'Whether the outbreak is one of Ebola, or Zika, or another infectious agent, health authorities scramble to communicate with their diverse publics about elements of risk, decisional choices, and actions required. With the advent of real-time digital media platforms, social media outlets, and ubiquitous mobile devices, the public dynamically participates in the co-creation of what constitutes risk, for whom, with what consequence, and requiring what action. This co-creation is a complex, dynamic, and emergent process, and this book provides invaluable insights, among many, into how "wisdom of the crowd" can be harnessed in ways that can spell the difference between life and death. A must read for those interested in the interface of infectious disease, communicating risk, and the potential and pitfalls of social media.'

*Arvind Singhal, Ph.D. Marston Endowed Professor of Communication, University of Texas at El Paso and Professor, Hedmark University of Applied Sciences, Norway*

'Ground-breaking – if only this work had been available, understood and applied in early 2014 at the beginning of the West African Ebola epidemic both the human toll in lives lost and the excesses of the following Fearbola events could have been significantly curtailed. In such outbreaks when vaccines and effective counter-measures are not yet available, effective communication is our strongest asset and by drawing on the combined informed input of the "public" we can better insure optimization of these public health interventions. This work should be required reading for medical and media professionals alike.'

*James J. James, M.D., Executive Director, Society for Disaster Medicine and Public Health and Adjunct Professor, University of Georgia, USA*

'The authors take a controversial position on controversies regarding scientific evidence, namely, that lay skepticism about scientists' claims is not always indefensible. Paying particular attention to the role of new media, the authors take a broad perspective in asking how the public and the experts can achieve warranted mutual respect, recognizing the commonalities and conflicts in their interests. The authors pursue that question vigorously, drawing broadly on academic research from social science and the humanities, illustrated with engaging historical and topical examples.'

*Baruch Fischhoff, Ph.D., Howard Heinz University Professor, Carnegie Mellon University*

'The essence of this book is splendidly embedded in its title, which suggests, with a subtle play of words, that new media are modifying "communication" of infectious diseases. Infectious diseases are indeed communicable in two senses, because they can be transmitted and because they are spoken. The authors wisely introduce the reader into metaphors surrounding infectious diseases and the way in which new media are shaping them. This is a great, fascinating, book, which raises critical questions about health risk communication and helps us re-think many current, obsolete, standards.'

*Emilio Mordini, M.D., Responsible Technology, France; chair of the Risk Communication working party of the Collaborative Management Platform for Detection and Analyses of (Re-)emerging and Foodborne Outbreaks in Europe (COMPARE)*

D0139976

# Risk Communication and Infectious Diseases in an Age of Digital Media

In a digital world where the public's voice is growing increasingly strong, how can health experts best exert influence to contain the global spread of infectious diseases? Digital media sites provide an important source of health information. At the same time, they also serve as powerful platforms for the public to air personal experiences and concerns, and have led to "scientific skepticism" – a growing phenomenon of civil skepticism towards various scientific topics, particularly health issues under dispute, characterized by uncertainty. Such issues tend to surface often during Emerging Infectious Diseases (EID) outbreaks and epidemics.

Following the shift in the role of the public from recipients to a vocal entity, this book explores the different organizational strategies for communicating public health information and identifies common misconceptions that can inhibit effective communication with the public. Drawing on original research and a range of global case studies, this timely volume offers an important assessment of the complex dynamics at play in managing risk and informing public health decisions.

Providing thought-provoking analysis of the implications for future health communication policy and practice, this book is primarily suitable for academics and graduate students interested in understanding how public health communication has changed. It may also be useful to healthcare professionals.

**Anat Gesser-Edelsburg** is a senior lecturer, the head of the Health Promotion department at the School of Public Health and the founding director of the Health and Risk Communication Research Center at University of Haifa Israel.

**Yaffa Shir-Raz** is a senior health journalist, a health and risk communication researcher at the University of Haifa, and a lecturer in Sammy Ofer School of Communication, IDC Herzliya, Israel.

# Routledge Studies in Public Health

# Risk Communication and Infectious Diseases in an Age of Digital Media

**Anat Gesser-Edelsburg and Yaffa Shir-Raz**

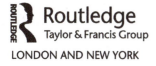

Routledge
Taylor & Francis Group

LONDON AND NEW YORK

First published 2017 by Routledge

2 Park Square, Milton Park, Abingdon, Oxfordshire OX14 4RN
52 Vanderbilt Avenue, New York, NY 10017

*Routledge is an imprint of the Taylor & Francis Group, an informa business*

First issued in paperback 2019

*British Library Cataloguing in Publication Data*
A catalogue record for this book is available from the British Library

*Library of Congress Cataloging in Publication Data*
Names: Gasser-Edelsburg, Anat, 1972- author. | Shir-Raz, Yaffa, author.
Title: Risk communication and infectious diseases in an age of digital
media / Anat Gesser-Edelsburg and Yaffa Shir-Raz.
Other titles: Routledge studies in public health.
Description: Abingdon, Oxon ; New York, NY : Routledge, 2017. | Series:
Routledge studies in public health | Includes bibliographical references
and index.
Identifiers: LCCN 2016025546| ISBN 9781138186064 (hardback) |
ISBN 9781315644073 (ebook)
Subjects: | MESH: Health Communication--trends | Health Information
Management--methods | Communicable Diseases, Emerging |
Communications Media
Classification: LCC R119.9 | NLM WA 590 | DDC 610.285--dc23
LC record available at https://lccn.loc.gov/2016025546

ISBN: 978-1-138-18606-4 (hbk)
ISBN: 978-0-367-22405-9 (pbk)

Typeset in Times New Roman
by Taylor & Francis Books

This book is dedicated to my beloved late mother, Nehama, whom I miss so much. To my father Yaacov and grandmother, Raya Lazar, my daughters, Lihi and Lev, my husband and true partner, Roni, and to all the Gessers and Edelsburgs. (Anat Gesser-Edelsburg)

To my husband shimon and my daughters Jasmin and Offir, who give me the courage to go forward with my dreams, to my beloved mother, Zipora, and in memory of my dearest father, Nachum. (Yaffa Shir-Raz)

The word "risk" derives from the early Italian risicare, which means "to dare". In this sense, risk is a choice rather than a fate. The actions we dare to take, which depend on how free we are to make choices, are what the story of risk is all about. And that story helps define what it means to be a human being.

(Bernstein, 1998)

# Contents

# Acknowledgement

As we end the long and intriguing journey of writing this book, we would like to express our thanks and deep appreciation to Ed Needle and Catherine Gray, Health and Social Care list former Senior Editors, who believed in our book, read through the first chapters and made useful suggestions, which greatly improved the exposition. Special thanks go to Grace McInnes, Health and Social Care list Senior Editor, Carolina Antunes, the Editorial Assistant, Siobhán Greaney, our book production editor, and Susan Dunsmore the book's editor, for their efficient guidance and patient assistance through the production process to publication, and to Louisa Vahtrick, who helped us through the administration.

The research leading to some of the results presented in this book, received funding from the European Union Seventh Framework Programme under grant agreements no. HEALTH-F3-2012-278723 (TELL ME) and no. SCIENCE-IN-SOCIETY-2013-1-612236.

# Introduction
## The Transformation of Emerging Infectious Disease Communication in the New Media Age

### Scientific skepticism: a growing phenomenon of citizen skepticism regarding health issues in dispute

The Zika Virus, Ebola, H1N1, MERS, polio and SARS outbreaks, as well as the HPV and measles vaccines, are issues that have been at the center of medical disputes in recent years. Time and again, in crisis situations caused by disease outbreaks, the importance of Emerging Infectious Disease (EID) communication resurfaces. Yet, as the *New York Times* medical journalist Lawrence Altman has argued, "even though health officials have had ample time – years – to polish their language skills" and lots of practice, they still failed to communicate important health information in response to the Ebola epidemic in 2014, just as they did during the HIV crisis in the 1980s. And so, as he put it, "history repeats itself" (Ratzan and Moritsugu, 2014). This failure is surprising, especially in light of the vast developments in the field of risk communication and the growing understanding of its importance during pandemic outbreaks. As Barry (2009, p. 324) noted, following the communication crises surrounding the successive outbreaks of Mad Cow Disease, SARS, and H1N1: "In the next influenza pandemic, be it now or in the future, be the virus mild or virulent, the single most important weapon against the disease will be a vaccine. The second most important will be communication."

So why, despite awareness of the importance of risk communication, are there glaring gaps between health organizations and the public? To address this important question, we must take an empirical approach that takes into account the enormous changes that have occurred in the public sphere during the 21st century. Although extensive literature exists on EID communication, most of it is still theoretical and has not addressed the role of new media in changing and designing the new public sphere. This book will attempt to address these gaps. To that end, we devote special attention to the technological revolution of the digital age, which has engendered a social revolution and led to what is known as "the wisdom of the crowd" – the collective wisdom that shapes societies and nations, economics, and policies today.

In this context, we propose coining the term "scientific skepticism." In the risk communication literature, and especially in the work focusing on vaccines, the term "vaccination refusers" has long been used to describe parents who raise doubts or questions regarding vaccine efficacy and safety. However, accumulating studies and data reveal that while many parents do (rationally) evaluate the benefits and risks of vaccines (Velan, 2011; Velan et al., 2012), and as a result tend to delay vaccination for their children or refuse selected vaccines – direct and absolute opposition to vaccination is rare (CDC, 2013; Velan, 2011). The term "vaccination hesitancy" articulates this dilemma (Diekema, 2012; Healy and Pickering, 2011; Smith and Marshall, 2010; Velan et al., 2012).

Unlike "vaccination refusal," or even "vaccination hesitancy," the term "scientific skepticism" expresses the idea that in fact, these are not marginal groups, but rather a growing phenomenon of civil skepticism towards various scientific topics, particularly health issues under dispute and characterized by uncertainty. Such issues tend to surface often during EID outbreaks and epidemics. The public's scientific skepticism addresses not only vaccines, but is a widespread phenomenon, encompassing a variety of health issues and means of disease prevention, as seen, for example, in the case of the Ebola epidemic. To ignore this fact, while labeling the skeptic public as extremists, would mean burying our heads in the sand.

This book seeks to explore controversial issues in the context of EID outbreaks that expose the roots of the gaps between health authorities and the public, and to examine how the public understands science. It makes suggestions regarding how organizations should cope with the wisdom of the crowd, as expressed in social media.

The new media have become an important source of health information and a platform for discussing personal experiences, opinions, and concerns regarding illnesses and treatments, and have contributed to the shift in the role of the public from being recipients to an active and vocal entity. This fundamental shift has created challenges for health organizations, and led to a paradox that must be addressed. On one hand, both the public and the organizations have influence within the public sphere, and the official health organizations are no longer the main source of information. On the other hand, the experts – doctors and health professionals – still have to manage the crisis. This book will raise a crucial question: In a reality in which the public sphere gives laypeople increasing influence, how can organizations respect the power emanating from them, while still exerting influence based on their professional knowledge and expertise, in order to manage the outbreak?

In order to deal with the paradox that the organizations face, the second factor – the public – must be added into the equation. This book will explore the tension between how the public is perceived by the authorities – as ignorant, acting based on emotions, anxiety, and prejudice – versus how the public perceives itself. We will examine the public's sources of information; what people want to know, and to what extent. We ask: What are the public's needs and risk perceptions, and do they really act out of panic during outbreaks? Does the public want to receive information that includes uncertainty? How do people make decisions? How do they understand science? How do they combine science with experience?

These central questions encompasses a number of issues, which will be addressed in detail in the book. For instance, what challenges and dilemmas do organizations face in this new public sphere? What are the different strategies used by the organizations to communicate information? What are the organizational policies and practices? What is the real purpose underlying the organizations' risk communication?

The book will also address the role of journalists and doctors in the communication circuit: are journalists doing their job as the watchdogs of democracy? How do the new media affect their work? What is the role of physicians in risk communication?

## The structure of the book

To address the issues raised above, the book presents seven chapters about the aforementioned stakeholders: the organizations, the mediators, and the public.

Chapter 1 will examine "The Public Sphere and Health Communication in the Context of Emergent Infectious Diseases," and will try to explain the psychological and cultural basis of the public sphere in the context of epidemics. The first part of the chapter goes back in time and looks at historic memory of epidemics and vaccines. In ancient times, epidemics served in literature, drama, and art as a metaphor for society's ills. The modern world led to a dramatic change in humanity's ability to cope with epidemics, and the transition from relying on God to relying on science gave rise to the new force embodied in the redeeming instrument of vaccination. This led a tremendous health revolution, but can also be said to have sown the seeds of skepticism, worsened by the misuse of risk communication by governments, which we will expand upon throughout the book.

The second part of the chapter focuses on the public sphere in the context of pandemics. It examines the role of the organizations in the age of new media. The organizations' understanding that coping with an epidemic crisis should occur by situating the public sociologically and psychologically has led to changes regarding the role of communication in crisis management. There has been much progress since the predominance of the principle of the "hypodermic needle," where the public was "injected" with the message. There are several models that during crises focus on active communication, situating the public at the center and viewing it as an active partner and not merely a recipient of data. This repositioning of the public as an active participant is facilitated by new mobile technologies, especially smartphones and Internet-based tools. The call for the "engagement" of the public is a concept which still reflects a passive audience to be engaged, and does not take into account the polyvocality of the public and a reality in which the opinions and knowledge of the public "compete" with those of the health authorities. Moreover, the understanding that the public in the 21st century is a full partner necessitates a greater understanding of the social and technological realms in which the public operates. With this in mind, Chapter 1 addresses the challenges that organizations face when communicating in the public sphere. We will do this by introducing a theory-driven holistic framework that portrays the reality of outbreak communication in the age of new media and shows how the organizations communicate risk to the public in this reality (Gesser-Edelsburg et al., 2015). Our framework is not based on a hierarchic, linear structure. Rather, it is circular and multi-directional, corresponding to a complex and constantly changing reality. Throughout the book, we will point out existing gaps.

Chapter 2 treats "The Challenge of Digital Media for Health Organizations." Before the technological age, people used sources of information from their immediate environment, and officials were the exclusive source of authority. The Internet changed the rules of the game and increased the public's activism, expressed by its searching for, sharing, and distributing information. The public's empowerment led the organizations to recognize the importance of the Internet sphere and the public's needs. Nevertheless, Chapter 2 indicates that, despite that recognition, the old spirit of the organizations still haunts the public sphere on the social media.

Chapter 3 will focus on "Organizational Policy and Practice." The authorities' policy regarding infectious diseases manifests in how they operate in three domains: the law, education, and ethics. Chapter 3 will examine how authorities operate in these three domains over the long term, and will emphasize the organizations' tendency over the years to neglect the educational aspect and focus on vaccine policies. In addition, it examines whether in countries that do not have mandatory vaccination policies, the authorities actually conduct a true dialog with the public, or only do so as a pretense for a patronizing policy instrument.

Chapter 4 will discuss organizations' "Strategies for Communicating Health Information and Risk." This chapter includes different communications strategies or framings employed by the organizations in order to promote their policy. Framing effect refers to the change in attitudes, emotions or behavior resulting from different representations of information. Message framing is central in the context of pandemics. Language and terminology are crucial, since they affect the decision-making process of social judgments and actions. Chapter 4 will demonstrate how the strategic framing of truth and falsehood is transformed into myths, how the scientific discourse is reduced to certainty, and how an epidemic turns into a problem that begs a solution. We will present examples of various frames used by organizations in order to portray vaccines – including controversial ones, in terms of efficacy and/or safety – as the ultimate solution.

In addition, Chapter 4 will demonstrate how the discourse preserves control mechanisms using statistical methodologies. We will raise a question usually not asked directly in studies focusing on infectious diseases: Is the purpose of risk communication to help the public make decisions or to make the public vaccinate? This question is of great importance to risk communication. We will examine how in various outbreaks and epidemics, getting people to vaccinate was the organizations' explicit purpose, while helping the public make decisions was sometimes a marginal or neglected aim.

Chapter 5 will examine "The Role of Health Journalists and Medical Experts." These two stakeholders play a central role in mediating and communicating the risks to the public. The obvious assumption is that in democratic countries the public views them as expressing its concerns. The question raised in this chapter is whether and how they do their jobs, and if the sometimes symbiotic relationships that develop between the industry and organizations and the stakeholders affect the way they communicate risk. The chapter will present examples of this dilemma and discuss its potential ramifications, stemming from the pharmaceutical industry's influence on the way journalists and doctors function.

Chapter 6 will address "The Public's Understanding and Decision-Making Regarding Science and Risk." The chapter will focus on two issues: (1) How do people make decisions in crises; and (2) what do they expect from the authorities? The chapter will illustrate the shift from early theories of risk communication that focused on persuading the public by lifting so-called irrational barriers, by presenting accurate, credible, and scientific information, to the current literature-based theories that show people make decisions based on their evaluation of the relevance of the risk to their lives. The public's behavior during crises may be driven by contradictory motives, such as rationality with emotion (Slovic et al., 2004), or seeking official sources of security while tending to think independently.

Contrary to what we know from the literature, some authorities continue to adhere to myths about the public's decision-making process. This chapter will examine two common myths maintained by some decision-makers: the first is that in crises the public panics, and in order not to strengthen that "tendency," it needs to be given brief instructions with selective information. The second myth is that because the public is not professional, it does not understand or know how to process scientific information. This chapter will examine the second myth in light of two opposing approaches – the information deficit model (Dickson, 2005) and citizen science (Irwin, 1995).

The first approach distinguishes between experts, who have the information, and non-experts, who lack information and understanding, and are in some way ignorant of the scientific knowledge about risk and probability. In contrast, the second approach – Citizen Science – is much more optimistic about the public's knowledge and does not view the public versus the experts in dichotomous terms, but rather argues that both experts and the public understand and interpret information based on cultural, moral, and emotional backgrounds (Waddell, 1995). According to this approach, not only does the public have scientific knowledge, but it is important to involve the public in building intervention programs. We will examine these two conflicting approaches in light of several empirical studies we have conducted, in which we analyzed the public's attitudes and opinions on Facebook, Twitter, and online forums during various crises.

Chapter 7 will present "Observations and Lessons: Managing Health Risks in the Age of Digital Media." The conceptual framework presented in Chapter 1 describes how ideally, organizations should embrace the public. In order to turn that metaphoric embrace into practical directives for health organizations in the virtual age, Chapter 7 will discuss the question of how organizations manage the scientific discourse, and then point out the specific challenges they face when dealing with the scientific discourse in the technological sphere. In addition, we present possible management ideas. We will propose recommendations for how to transcend two-way communication in creating a dialog with the public through an emergency knowledge management system, based on building a community presence on the social media when a crisis is imminent.

## References

Barry, J. M. (2009). Pandemics: Avoiding the mistakes of 1918. *Nature*, 459(7245), 324–325.

CDC (2013). Vaccination coverage among children in kindergarten – United States, 2012–2013 school year. Available at: www.cdc.gov/mmwr/preview/mmwrhtml/mm6230a3.htm

Dickson, D. (2005). The case for a 'deficit model' of science communication. *SciDev.Net*. Available at: www.scidev.net/global/communication/editorials/the-case-for-a-deficit-model-of-science-communic.html (accessed April 24, 2016).

Diekema, D. S. (2012). Issues leading to vaccine hesitancy. Paper presented at the Meeting 2 of the Institute of Medicine Committee on the Assessment of Studies of Health Outcomes Related to the Recommended Childhood Immunization Schedule.

Gesser-Edelsburg, A., Shir-Raz, Y., Walter, N., *et al.* (2015). The public sphere in emerging infectious disease communication: Recipient or active and vocal partner? *Disaster Medicine and Public Health Preparedness*, 9(4), 447–458.

Healy, C. M., and Pickering, L. K. (2011). How to communicate with vaccine-hesitant parents. *Pediatrics*, 127(suppl. 1), S127–S133.

Irwin, A. (1995). *Citizen Science: A Study of People, Expertise and Sustainable Development*. London: Routledge.

Ratzan, S. C., and Moritsugu, K. P. (2014). Ebola crisis: Communication chaos we can avoid. *Journal of Health Communication*, 19(11), 1213–1215.

Slovic, P., Finucane, M., Peters, E., and MacGregor, D. (2004). Risk as analysis and risk as feelings: Some thoughts about affect, reason, risk and rationality. *Risk Analysis*, 24(2), 311–322.

Smith, M. J., and Marshall, G. S. (2010). Navigating parental vaccine hesitancy. *Pediatric Annals*, 39(8), 476–482.

Velan, B. (2011). Acceptance on the move: Public reaction to shifting vaccination realities. *Human Vaccines*, 7(12), 1261–1270.

Velan, B., Boyko, V., Lerner-Geva, L., Ziv, A., Yagar, Y., and Kaplan, G. (2012). Individualism, acceptance and differentiation as attitude traits in the public's response to vaccination. *Human Vaccines and Immunotherapeutic*, 8(9), 1272–1282.

Waddell, C. (1995). Defining sustainable development: A case study in environmental communication. *Technical Communication Quarterly*, 4(2), 201–216.

# 1 The Public Sphere and Health Communication in the Context of Emergent Infectious Diseases

## Part 1 Historic memory of epidemics and vaccines

Desperate in view of the mounting death toll, which by August 1577 had reached around 10,000 (Cohn Jr, 2010), the people of Milan vowed to build a temple and dedicate it Saint Sebastian if he succeeded in purging the curse of the Black Death from their city. Saint Sebastian was the patron saint of plague. It was believed that the plague of 680 that had struck northern Italy nearly a thousand years earlier, had stopped only after a relic of the saint's arm was moved from Rome and set up in the Church of San Pietro in Vincoli in Pavia. The foundation stone of the new temple in Milan was laid in September 1577, and on January 20, 1578, on the Feast of Saint Sebastian, the plague was officially declared to have passed. To this day, the cylindrical temple, located near Milan's Duomo, symbolizes pain and rebirth from darkness and death.

In Bristow's book, *American Pandemic: The Lost Worlds of the 1918 Influenza Epidemic* (2012), the author argues that the Americans have developed a "national amnesia," erasing the dark days of pandemic from their collective memory, in order to compose an optimistic narrative. Yet, the echoes of the great epidemics and the death they entail are never really erased from our collective memory. They may indeed be buried deep in the storerooms of our mind, but just as the Milanese brought back the memory of an ancient plague in 1577 that had struck nearly a thousand years earlier to help them cope with the new incidence of the plague, we revive memories of previous epidemics each time a new one strikes.

### Epidemics as a metaphor for societal ills

While other illnesses that have killed and disabled many millions, such as malaria, can be explained as an inevitable part of poor living conditions, an epidemic is a disease that literally "falls upon people" (in Greek, *epi* means "upon or above," and *demos* means "people") (Cunningham, 2008). It strikes indiscriminately and is by definition episodic and unpredictable. As a result, epidemics are highly visible and much more frightening, and thus have a special cultural salience (Rosenberg, 2008).

Memories of previous epidemics are expressed in various and diverse cultural representations. They are depicted in many historical monuments and architectural creations throughout the world, in paintings, in sculptures, in engravings and in photography, and rendered through music and dancing. They are also present in literature, as well as in theater and cinema (Vidal et al., 2007). Epidemics, as they are articulated in all these artistic expressions, symbolize our sense of helplessness in the face of uncertainty and death, as well as the arbitrary nature of death itself. More importantly, they can be seen as a mirror of society's internal chaos– the social, political, even theological ills. The heroes of many works that portray epidemics are in many cases healers, who, with their therapeutic talent, compassion and altruism, try to fight evil or treat the sick.

One pre-eminent example is *The Plague* by Albert Camus, which tells the story of a plague that strikes the Algerian city of Oran, and of the collective response to the catastrophe. It is believed that the novel is based on a real event – the great cholera epidemic in 1849, which killed a large percentage of the population of Oran (Mitchell, 2012). Yet, the novel, published in 1947 – in the wake of World War II, can be read as an allegory symbolizing the ills of a society infected with complacency, evil, and denial, and of human suffering in an indifferent world. Its heroes, Dr. Rieux and his friends Tarrou and Grand doggedly battle the plague, rebelling against the senselessness of death. Despite the knowledge that the disease is incurable, Dr. Rieux does not abandon his patients, providing them with care and exceptional compassion.

Another example that connects the ancient and the modern world is Connie Willis' novel *Doomsday Book* (Willis, 1992). The story takes place England in both the mid-21st century, and the 14th century. Due to the collapse of the time travel coordinates for her trip, the protagonist, Kivrin Engle, a time-traveling historian, is caught in a small medieval village in England during the Black Death epidemic in 1348, hoping to be rescued by her colleagues from Oxford of the 2050s. Eventually, the epidemic strikes the modern world and threatens it. The significance of the story is clear: the time traveler is a heroine who struggles to unify two different and yet similar worlds.

Homer's *Iliad* also incorporates reference to an epidemic. The first poem describes how Apollo, furious at King Agamemnon for refusing to return his priest's daughter, sends a fatal plague upon the Greek army, causing the death of many soldiers: "a plague sent down by the lines of his arch."

In *The Decameron*, Giovanni Boccaccio's most famous literary work (Boccaccio, 1973), the plague is used as a satiric metaphor to expose the injustices and crimes of various religions. The book is a collection of stories, whose depictions of sexuality, lust, and betrayal criticize religion and clergymen.

In the theater, perhaps the most famous play describing an epidemic is *Oedipus the King*, Sophocles' tragedy. Following a vicious murder, a lethal plague strikes the city of Thebes. Plants, animals, and people are all dying. Devoted to his people, Oedipus tirelessly tries to find the cause of the plague. Tragically, as his investigation progresses, he discovers the bitter truth – the failure of his attempts to fight his destiny and prevent the fulfillment of the prophecy according to which he was supposed to kill his own father and marry his mother, and so he himself was cause of the plague. Thus, the plague serves as a catalyst for identifying Oedipus' original sin. It is a metaphorical expression of the inner plague in Oedipus' soul.

In many creations related to the Black Death, a central motif which was popular in the late-medieval period is the Dance of Death (in French: *La Danse Macabre*), in which skeletons who represent death force the living to dance with them (Christian, 2011). The Dance of Death has both literary and visual representations in drama, poetry, music, paintings, engravings, and sculptures. Its purpose is to remind viewers and readers of the universality of death and of their own mortality (Oosterwijk, 2009, 2012). Striking examples include Hans Holbein's woodcuts, first published in 1538 (Byrne, 2006), and the "Imago mortis," a woodcut made in 1493 by the German painter and printmaker, Michael Wolgemut, inspired by the horrors of the Black Plague (Oosterwijk, 2012). Wolgemut, like Holbein and many others who portray the Dance of Death, illustrates the figure of death encroaching on life. Just as in ancient and modern books, novels and poems, the epidemic unifies past and present, the inside and the outside world. Death is indiscriminate, striking both young and old, the poor and the rich, nobles and commoners, and all of them, regardless of class, gender or religion, join the Dance of Death in awe.

In the cinema, Vidal, Tibaruenc and Gonzalez (Vidal et al., 2007) identify 100 films that portray infectious diseases. Well-known examples include *Death in Venice* (Luchino Visconti, 1971), which represented a cholera epidemic; *The Seventh Seal* (Ingmar Bergman, 1957), portraying the Black Plague; and *Outbreak* (Wolfgang Petersen, 1995), featuring an Ebola-like virus. Pappas, Seitaridis, Akritidis, and Tsianos (2003) reviewed films focusing on epidemics, and found that most of them focus on the threat presented by outbreaks. Among the films they reviewed are *1918* (Ken Harrison, 1985), which focused on the 1918 influenza epidemic; *Gypsy Fury* (Christian Jacques, 1949), which described the Black Death; *Trollsyn* (Ola Solum, 1994) and *Dr. Bull* (John Ford, 1933) – two films that portrayed typhoid epidemics.

All of these films represent an attempt to find a way to deal with the lack of control and the uncertainty that characterize epidemics. For example, in *Death in Venice*, the main character, Gustav von Aschenbach, struggles with an overwhelming attraction to a 14-year-old boy. In *The Seventh Seal*, the hero embarks on an inner journey in view of the raging epidemic, and searches his soul, while the characters struggle with passion and fantasies.

Thus, many artists, in various fields of art, have chosen to use epidemics and their unpredictable, threatening, and devastating power to articulate the destructiveness within human society. In many works, the epidemic symbolizes the social consciousness of evil and death and the struggle against them.

The memories of previous epidemics are also very prominent in the mass media. Each time a new outbreak strikes, the news is inundated with stories of past pandemics. The most recent example is the Ebola epidemic in West

Africa. In October 2014, after the death of Thomas Eric Duncan, the first Ebola patient to be diagnosed on US soil (Fernandez and Philipps, 2014), articles on deadly epidemics appeared in almost every media outlet (Bergen, 2014; Branato, 2015; Moore, n.d.; National Geographic Staff, 2014). Similar articles appeared during the H1N1 pandemic (Dominus, 2009; MacKenzie and Marshall, 2009).

### Dealing with epidemics: From reliance on God to vaccine development

> But the hand of the Lord was heavy upon them of Ashdod, and he destroyed them, and smote them with tumors, even Ashdod and the coasts thereof.
>
> (1 Samuel 5:6)

For thousands of years, epidemics were perceived as a manifestation of divine vengeance – a punishment inflicted by God for sins committed by humans. In the Hebrew Bible, the First Book of Samuel describes how the Philistines, having captured the Ark of the Covenant from the Israelites, suffered an out-break of "tumors" (Hebrew, *ophal*), which followed them as they moved the Ark of the Covenant from city to city. Evaluating the events in this ancient story, some modern scholars suggest that the disaster the Philistines suffered could have been an epidemic of some kind, probably a plague (Freemon, 2005; Griffin, 2000). This is reinforced by the unexpected event described later in the chapter – soon after the Philistines return the Ark of the Covenant, the plague ravaged the Israelites, killing many of them, just as it had the Philistines. Yet, the Philistines believed the disease was inflicted by the God of Israel (verses 10–12) – a punishment inflicted by a God mightier than their own for having transgressed against Him. Aware of Israelite history, they recalled the heavy price Pharaoh and his people had paid for their refusal to release the Israelites – they suffered from plague and vermin infestations (Exodus 9:8–15). Thus, they hoped that returning the Ark to its rightful owner would appease God (De Paolo, 2006). Similarly, during the Justinian Plague in 540, the Byzantine historian Procopius of Caesarea blamed the outbreak on the emperor, declaring him either a demon or a sinner punished by God (Horgan, 2014).

This perception of epidemics as inflicted by God as punishment persisted for many centuries, and was believed even by learned physicians (Cunningham, 2008). The only way to counter this "punishment" was to plead for God's mercy through prayer and fasting (Cunningham, 2008), or to designate scapegoats, such as foreigners, beggars, pilgrims, lepers and especially the Jews (Levack, 1995; Vidal et al., 2007). The search for scapegoats reached its climax during the 14th century, as the Black Death swept across Europe, fomenting anxiety and despair that prevailed, especially in view of the unprecedented scope and magnitude of the plague (Moore, 2007; Nirenberg, 1996). Jews were blamed for deliberately causing the disease by poisoning the wells (Foa, 2000; Levy, 2005). Starting in 1348, many Jewish communities were attacked and their inhabitants massacred or burned alive. Persecution spread across Europe

(Foa, 2000). Witches were another group who werre persecuted because they were accused of spreading the plague. Christian (2011) argues that the plague of 1348 was a factor that contributed to the intensity of the witch hunts that occurred between 1550 and 1650.

Nevertheless, in the Middle Ages, a transformation began. The recurrence of the Black Death and the horrific magnitude of the plague led to a feeling of disillusionment with the Church. Thus, the blind acceptance of the plague as a punishment was replaced by a different understanding of epidemics as a part of the natural world, and this allowed for the possibility for human intervention (Dolber, 2010). As time passed and the plague recurred, people shifted from religious means to medical aid for prevention and treatment (Cohn, 2002). Well aware of their own helplessness against the plague, medieval doctors did not completely turn their backs on religion, but rather bridged the divine and the natural, combining faith in God with a variety of earthly treatment regimens. These included, as the French physician and surgeon Guy de Chauliac wrote in his treatise *Chirurgia Magna*, "pills, to diminish the blood by phlebotomy"; fire "to purify the air"; "theriac" (a medical concoction) "to strengthen the heart"; "fruits and good-smelling things"; fleeing to a non-infected area, and other preventive and treatment measures (Wallis, 2010, p. 421).

In 1348, when the Black Death struck France, King Philip VI commissioned the Faculty of Medicine of Paris to write a report on the plague and make recommendations. The document they wrote offered both a diagnosis and a management plan. Although drawing on astrological explanations – "the conjunction of Mars and Jupiter caused a great pestilence in the air, especially when they come together in a hot, wet sign, as was the case in 1345," and acknowledging that their work was carried out "with God's help," the report reflected a deep faith in the human mind and ability to comprehend and thus control the catastrophe (Wallis, 2010, p. 421). Subsequently, in 1365, John of Burgundy, a French physician, wrote one of the most thorough medical books on the prevention and cure of plague. Burgundy theorized about causes of the plague and explained how to prevent it, incorporating his past experience and faith in God's help (Zahler, 2009).

Gradually, European governments understood that individual measures alone would not suffice to contain the plague. In Italy, the Great City Council of Ragusa passed a law in 1377 establishing a mandatory isolation period of 30 days for citizens or visitors from plague-endemic areas who sought to enter the city (Stuard, 1992). In time, the isolation period was extended from 30 to 40 days – or from *trentino* to *quarantine* – a term derived from the Italian *quaranta*, meaning "forty" (Mackowiak and Sehdev, 2002; Stuard, 1992), from which the English word "quarantine" is derived. This word is still used to describe the practice of isolating people who have been exposed to a contagious disease to see if they become sick (Mackowiak and Sehdev, 2002). During the following 80 years, similar laws were introduced in Marseilles, Venice, Pisa, and Genoa (Mackowiak & Sehdev, 2002; Matovinovic, 1969). In 1540, when the plague recurred in Vienna, the medical faculty of the city authored a treatise, which "was widely distributed and contained two orders: streets must be cleaned twice weekly, and aromatic wood must be burned in order to improve the air of the city" (Velimirovic and Velimirovic, 1989, p. 817).

In 1546, the Italian doctor, poet, and scholar Giromalo Fracastoro published his theory of contagion, *Decontagione et contagiosis morbis et eorum curatione*, proposing that epidemics are caused by tiny particles from outside the body – "seeds of disease," that may be passed on and transmit infection by direct or indirect contact or even from a distance (Nutton, 1990). This emphasis on "seeds of disease" as an explanation for the plague and typhus preceded the microbial theory of diseases by three centuries (Bartlett, 2005).

At about the same time that European doctors were struggling to understand the causes of the Black Death to find a cure, in China, physicians began practicing variolation to prevent smallpox. Smallpox is a deadly disease that has killed millions of people throughout the world since its appearance around 3,000 years ago (WHO, 2015). The practice, based on exposing healthy people to tissue or fluid from the scabs caused by the disease (NHS, 2016), is thought to have been first introduced in China in the 16th century (Leung, 1996), although some argue that it was carried out as early as the 10th century (Needham, 1980). It was implemented using several methods, including inserting a piece of cotton covered with pus or squama into the nostril, or, later on, in the 18th century, by using powdered squama blown into the nostril through a thin silver tube (Leung, 1996). In the Middle East, where variolation was also practiced, another method was used – by mixing the matter into a shallow incision on the arm made with a surgeon's needle (Grey, 2016). The individual who was variolated then contracted a mild form of smallpox, and upon recovery, was immune to the disease (NIH, 2013). The procedure was also practiced in Africa (Williams, 2010), Turkey, and Greece (Razzell, 1977), and eventually, it was introduced into Europe and North America in the early 18th century (Bonanni and Santos, 2011; Henderson, 2009; NHS, 2016).

Yet in Western Europe, variolation was first viewed with skepticism (Grey, 2016). In 1714, the Italian physician Emmanuel Timoni, a Fellow of the Royal Society, submitted a paper describing the procedure in detail, which was later published in the *Philosophical Transactions* (Adler, 2004). He argued that his 40 years of experience practicing variolation in Constantinople proved that this practice was immensely efficient in combating smallpox epidemics (Grey, 2016). Nevertheless, European physicians remained skeptical regarding the procedure and its efficacy and safety, and were reluctant to practice it themselves (Grey, 2016; Guerrini, 2003).

The individual thought to have contributed the most to acceptance of the practice of variolation by the medical establishment was Lady Mary Wortley Montagu, the wife of the British ambassador to the Ottoman Empire. Lady Montagu herself was a survivor of smallpox, left with massive scars on her face, and had lost her brother to the disease (Riedel, 2005). In 1717, she learned about the procedure in Constantinople (Fenner et al., 1988), and was so enthusiastic about it, she asked the embassy's surgeon doctor, Charles

Maitland, to inoculate her 5-year-old son, Edward, and later on, her 3-year-old daughter, Mary (Guerrini, 2003). Her enthusiasm caught the attention of Sir Hans Sloane, the king's physician. He wanted proof of the procedure's efficacy and safety. In 1721, he asked and received the king's permission to conduct an experiment: six prisoners from Newgate Prison in London were inoculated in exchange for their release. Five of the six developed smallpox, but all of them recovered, and were then released from prison (Guerrini, 2003). After skepticism was expressed in several newspapers and pamphlets, as well as by members of the medical community, one of the released prisoners, 19-year-old Elizabeth Harrison, was sent to nurse a smallpox victim. Vulnerable due to her class and gender, illiterate and unemployed, Harrison's consent was hardly informed or voluntary. Yet, her continued good health convinced some doctors that the procedure was effective, and they began inoculating their patients. The Princess of Wales announced that she would pay for the inoculation of all the orphans in St. James's Parish – a gesture which, it was claimed, was actually another experiment (Guerrini, 2003). Although the plan was not carried out, six orphans did undergo the experiment and after they too displayed successful results, the Princess of Wales was convinced, and Maitland variolated her two daughters (Guerrini, 2003; Riedel, 2005). The procedure then became popular among both aristocratic and common people in Europe (NIH, 2013; Riedel, 2005).

However, variolation was not risk-free. In 1783, Prince Octavius of Great Britain, the 4-year-old son of King George III, died a few days after being variolated (Baxby, 1984). Such deaths were not a rare occurrence. The overall mortality rate was estimated by authorities to be 1 in 200 (Baxby, 1984). Other risks included becoming infected with another epidemic or disease, such as syphilis, that could be transmitted by the procedure itself (Riedel, 2005). In addition, there was a chance that the mild form of the disease which the patient contracted would spread, causing an epidemic (NIH, 2013).

The first vaccine was introduced against this background. Folktales that dairymaids naturally infected with cowpox were immune to smallpox sparked the imagination of Edward Jenner, an English country doctor (Gross and Sepkowitz, 1998; Riedel, 2005). He speculated that deliberate infection with cowpox could cause immunity to smallpox (Riedel, 2005). On May 14, 1796, he conducted an experiment in which he collected the matter from fresh cowpox lesions on the arm of Sarah Nelms, a young dairymaid, and inoculated James Phipps, an 8-year-old boy. After a week, the boy complained of a pain in his armpit and two days later developed mild fever and a headache, from which he soon recovered. Six weeks later, Jenner inoculated James again, this time with pus from a human smallpox lesion. No disease developed, and Jenner concluded that immunity to smallpox was achieved (Case and Chung, 1997).

Jenner continued to experiment with inoculations using cowpox (Case and Chung, 1997). The book he wrote describing his findings, was first accepted by the medical community with mixed reviews, but was subsequently published and instantly attracted attention, becoming a bestseller in the medical community and among the London elite (Shurkin, 1979). The procedure then spread throughout England and even the USA through a chain of transmissions from individual to individual, usually orphans on board ships (NIH, 2013).

In 1804, Jenner was honored by Napoleon, who ordered compulsory vaccination in his army. In England, the Vaccination Act of 1853 mandated vaccination for infants (Daintith, 2008, p. 391), igniting vigorous opposition, not only of middle-class radical liberals, but also of working-class movements (Durbach, 2000).

Although for many years, Jenner was credited as the pioneer of smallpox vaccine and as the founder of immunization, he was neither the first to suggest the idea of using cowpox to achieve immunity against smallpox, nor the first to perform the practice. Several others, including Benjamin Jesty, had implemented it years before him (Gross and Sepkowitz, 1998; Riedel, 2005). Nevertheless, his work was the first scientific attempt to investigate the procedure (Riedel, 2005), and the story remains an inspiration to physicians fighting diseases that involve uncertainty (Wallis, 2010). In recognition of this early vaccine, the French physicist and chemist, Louis Pasteur (1822–1895), who established germ theory and developed the first vaccines for rabies and anthrax, coined the term "vaccine," from the Latin word for cow, *vacca* (Alexander, 2003).

Thus, the history of vaccine development abounds with heroic stories about visionaries who paved the way for the eradication or at the very least the dramatic reduction of many infectious diseases. Yet, this history is also riddled with stories describing unethical and sometimes immoral experiments such as those using orphans and prisoners, and with human tragedies that occurred following vaccinations, such as the death of Prince Octavius in 1783. Neither the heroic stories, nor those that invoke fear and anger are erased from our historic memory.

## Part 2 The public sphere in the context of pandemics

Collective memory embodies stories, images, fears, and desires. These are deeply embedded in the consciousness of the public sphere and influence how the public listens and reacts during an epidemic crisis. Building on this understanding, challenges faced by decision-makers during epidemics in the 21st century will be discussed. The book will examine what risk communication strategies are available to them, and how and to what extent they implement them.

The public sphere is critically important for modern societies. Its value lies in its ability to facilitate uninhibited and diverse discussion of public affairs. It presents a domain of social life in which public opinion is expressed, and issues relevant to the collective are communicated. Most contemporary conceptualizations of the public sphere are based on the ideas expressed by Jürgen Habermas in his book, *The Structural Transformation of the Public Sphere: An Inquiry into a Category of Bourgeois Society* (Habermas, 1989). According to Habermas, the public sphere is a neutral social space for critical debate among private persons who gather to discuss matters of common concern in a free and rational way. This sphere is open and accessible to the public. Habermas's public sphere is characterized by three major elements: (1) disregard of status (rejection of hierarchy); (2) the domain of common concern and interest; and (3) inclusivity (everyone must be able to participate) (Habermas, 1989). Thus, engagement within the public sphere according to Habermas, is blind to class differences and the connections between those active in the public sphere are formed through a mutual will to participate in matters of general interest.

Habermas argued that the new type of bourgeois public sphere that had emerged in Western Europe in the 18th century began to decline in the first half of the 20th century due to educational and capitalistic progress resulting in a stratified society with fewer mutual concerns. He pointed out that mass media contributed to the decay of the rational-critical discourse, turning the public sphere into a space in which the rhetoric and objectives of public relations and advertising are prioritized, and thus, into a vehicle for capitalist hegemony and ideological reproduction (Habermas, 2004).

Today, however, many media researchers, as well as political scientists and political activists, believe that the new media has given a renewed spirit to the concept of the public sphere, and that it has the potential to completely change societal communication (Jankowski and Van Selm, 2000; Van De Donk et al., 2004; Van Os et al., 2007). Indeed, the World Wide Web has become a domain in which all people can openly express and share concerns about broader societal issues. This is because it is widespread, and its infrastructure promises unregulated and unlimited discourse that operates beyond geographic boundaries.

### The paradox of the organizations

The public sphere in the 21st century has undergone a transformation generated by technological advances. The new media have become an important source of health information and a platform for discussing personal experiences, opinions, and concerns regarding illnesses and treatments, and have contributed to the shift in the role of the public from recipients to an active and vocal entity. This fundamental shift has led to a challenging paradox facing health orgnizations: On the one hand, both the public and the organizations have influence within the public sphere, and international health organizations are no longer the main sources of information. On the other hand, the experts – the doctors and health professionals – still have to manage crises. The question is how organizations can respect the power emanating from the public sphere, while still exerting influence, based on their professional knowledge and expertise in order to manage an outbreak.

As mentioned, one of the three main characteristics of Habermas's public sphere is the rejection of hierarchy and disregard of status (Habermas, 1989).

This means that in the public sphere, what health organizations say – even central organizations with international authority such as the World Health Organization (WHO) – can have the same influence as that of charismatic bloggers or other Internet users. Unofficial posts and blogs can have an influence equal to or greater than the assessments and recommendations of organizations. However, crises, such as pandemic outbreaks, present a challenge to the idea of the public sphere.

The organizations have the opportunity to enhance their rapport with the public through a dialog of equals. Yet they are still the ones who have the professional knowledge, authority and responsibility with which to manage the crisis (Thackeray et al., 2013). The question raised throughout this book is how that paradox works. Under these circumstances, in a sphere that gives power to the public, how can organizations act in a way that respects the public as equals, and yet expresses their professional knowledge and allows them to manage the outbreak?

The lessons learned during the SARS outbreak in 2002–2003 and the experience of communicating that crisis led the WHO to develop the *WHO Outbreak Communication Guidelines* (WHO, 2005). These guidelines stipulated that all acute public health event communications should be planned, organized, and executed according to five main principles: trust, announcing early, transparency, listening to the public, and planning (Härtl, 2013). Furthermore, the WHO has also conducted considerable training – both of its own and of health ministry staff worldwide – in the art of communicating quickly and effectively, according to the five principles established by the organization (Härtl, 2013). The UK plan (National Health Service, 2005) emphasizes the need to communicate regarding uncertainty; it offers advice and describes the constraints faced by the government in a pre-pandemic period; and in a pandemic period, states what information people will need and which actions they should take.

The UK plan also notes the importance of deeper public engagement, such as holding patient forums and focus groups to help identify public concerns, and having lay members on expert advisory groups. Similarly, in its discussion of risk communication in pandemic planning, Health Canada (2005) notes that the public would be more likely to take appropriate action during a crisis if they feel that they have been involved in the decision-making process. However, as Holmes (2008) has stated, the format of these emergency plans does not allow for elaboration on how such engagement is to be carried out; what issues, frustrations, and divisions might arise as a result of such engagement, and how it should be handled; and what formative qualitative research has been conducted.

Furthermore, most government reports have failed to break through the hierarchy barrier between the government and various publics, as indicated by current crises such as the Ebola outbreak. One of the main reasons is that social, economic and cultural gaps still exist in the global village that aspires to equality.

### Segmentation in the public sphere

Another basic condition which characterizes Habermas's public sphere is inclusivity, i.e., it has to be accessible to all participants, so that everyone can participate (Habermas, 1989). However, a precondition for accessibility to the discourse conducted in the public sphere is the ability to understand and make sense of it. To participate in the communication process, the information presented in it must be clear and understandable to all. People understand and interpret risks differently based on various factors, including gender, education level, income, culture, and ethnicity (Slovic, 2000).

Organizations must convince the public to adopt their messages about protective measures such as vaccines, and, in order to do so effectively, must tailor their messages according to socio-economic, cultural, educational and other contexts, rather than using "one-size fits all" messaging (Furgal et al., 2005; Krimsky and Plough, 1988; Lindell and Perry, 2004).

Indeed, international health authorities have addressed the subject of segmentation in their outbreak communication guidelines and reports (Gesser-Edelsburg et al., 2014). For example, the WHO's *International Health Regulations* (WHO, 2005) highlighted the importance of "taking into consideration the gender, sociocultural, ethnic or religious concerns of travelers" (WHO, 2008a). The 2008 edition of the *World Health Organization Outbreak Communication Planning Guide* stressed the need to "conduct an assessment of existing public communication capacity and existing research of community understanding, including demographics, literacy levels, language spoken as well as socio-economic and cultural backgrounds" (WHO, 2008b). The CDC's *Crisis and Emergency Risk Communication: Pandemic Influenza* recognized that "nonetheless, one size fits all never fits all people equally well" (Reynolds, 2007) and noted that it was important to "understand audience by age/culture/level of experience or familiarity with the subject/language/geographic location" (Reynolds, 2007). The idea of segmentation is also addressed in reports that have examined how the messages in the guidelines were conveyed to the public. These reports have indicated that special populations were targeted with specific prevention and control messages; key messages were provided to specific groups; and articles were targeted to specific audiences (Lam and McGreen, 2011).

Unfortunately, the theoretical foundation and understanding exemplified in guidelines and reports is not translated into practical "how to" recommendations at the local level, i.e., how exactly national health authorities should build segmented profiles of their various publics (Gesser-Edelsburg et al., 2014).

The gap between theory and practice is indeed evident when examining the local levels. At a Global Communications Conference, which took place in the midst of the H1N1 pandemic, countries were called on to adapt the communication strategies to their specific cultural needs (Brennan and Hall, 2009). The mere fact that this call was made points to a general lack of such cultural and social adaptation (Gesser-Edelsburg et al., 2014). Although government agencies have long recognized their responsibility to be sensitive to problems caused by "one-size fits all" messaging (Fischhoff, 2005), several studies have indicated that the idea of segmentation is still far from being implemented adequately. For example, an evaluation of how First Nations and Metis people in Manitoba, Canada responded to the public health management of the H1N1 pandemic, concluded that to better tailor both the messages and delivery, public health agencies need to devote more attention to the specific socio-economic, historical, and cultural contexts of such communities. This is because they are most at risk when planning for, communicating, and managing responses associated with pandemic outbreaks (Driedger et al., 2013). Similarly, evaluations of the risk communication practice during the H1N1 outbreak involving Pacific Peoples and Māori in New Zealand (Gray et al., 2012), Australian Aboriginal and Torres Strait Islanders (Massey et al., 2009; Massey et al., 2011; Rudge and Massey, 2010) concluded that more community-based information dissemination mechanisms are needed to avoid problems created by generic prevention and control messages.

These examples demonstrate that while the idea of segmentation is addressed in the international health authorities' guidelines and reports, the recognition of its importance still does not translate into practical recommendations. As a result, it does not occur at the local level, so that national authorities still use standardized and uniform messages and delivery channels for the diverse groups that comprise the public sphere. Moreover, in order for the campaigns to be tailored to communities, it is vital that the communities would perceive the program as such that suits their needs, and not only the agenda of the government or certain individuals. Organizations must take a "culturally-centered" approach (Dutta, 2007), with the aim of providing people with opportunities to express themselves and engage in critical dialog, allowing members of marginalized cultural groups to have their voices heard.

This approach of collaboration between organizations and different communities should be clarified and carried out before, during, and after the epidemic crisis, in order to establish trust between policymakers and the communities. In light of this, the challenges faced by organizations regarding the public sphere include building different profiles for different sub-populations, as each country has various sub-populations in its public sphere; tailoring communication and intervention plans to the needs of the different populations; and accepting communities' choices and decisions during the epidemic itself – which might possibly be the most difficult challenge. Are the organizations ready to accept the communities' own decisions during a crisis? And what does such acceptance mean in terms of public health?

### *How to treat the public's concerns*

Another central challenge faced by health organizations during outbreaks is how to acknowledge the public's anxiety and concerns. The gaps that remain in the field of emerging infectious disease communication are demonstrated by outbreaks such as H1N1 in 2009 and the recent Ebola crisis in Western Africa, indicating that basic tools are still needed. In the Ebola crisis, cases were first reported on February 9, 2014, yet the WHO did not declare an outbreak (Ministry of Health Republic of Botswana, 2014) until March 23 (WHO, 2014). Hence, for almost two months, there was hardly any news coverage or social media response. In addition, the overt messages delivered by health authorities regarding the risk degree contradicted the covert ones. The overt messages stated that the risk of contracting the disease was very low, stressing that the virus spreads mainly through direct contact with body fluids (Cassoobhoy 2014). However, articles described the two infected American aid workers who had returned to the USA and their admission into hospitals with special containment units (Achenbach et al., 2014). This sent a different message. This recent example and many others from various outbreaks indicate that there are still notable gaps between the degree of severity as perceived by the public and the actual severity.

According to Sandman (1989), risk perception is comprised of hazard plus outrage. The public's view of risk (as opposed to that of the experts) reflects not just the danger of the action (hazard), but also how they feel about the action and what emotions it produces (outrage). This means that other than the scientific aspect, feelings of outrage towards the risk must be considered. People associate high risk with issues towards which they have negative attitudes, regardless of the proved risk. Lack of agreement between experts and the public's perception of hazard and outrage can lead to controversy. Sandman maintains that one of the most important ways to deal with negative feelings of a population towards a certain issue is continuous communication with that population. The success of risk communication depends on the communicator's efforts to minimize the gap between the expert's risk assessment and the public's perceptions, in order to create mutual feedback between experts and the public (Fischhoff, 2004).

How organizations cope with anxiety and concerns is a critical issue in the public sphere, because it implies the need for the organization to take note of and appraise the public's collective memory concerning the epidemic, and the ensuing questions – Is this a known virus or a novel one? Are there any elements of uncertainty, and if yes, what is known about them? What are the issues in dispute between different experts? Does a vaccine exist? How safe is it? What is the collective memory associated with the vaccine?

Addressing the public's anxiety and concerns is a necessary condition for communicating the risk, as indicated by all of the professional literature on risk communication. However, it seems that organizations tend to fail in that respect time after time, by dismissing the public's anxiety and concerns about the epidemic (Maurice, 2015). In many countries, anxiety and concerns are still addressed on the ground by placating the public, mainly with the purpose of preventing the public from panicking, even though the theoretical literature indicates why that is problematic (Frewer et al., 2003; Sandman, 2007).

A respectful response to the anxiety and concerns of different publics might force the organization to reveal the "behind the scenes" activity of its deliberations, to expose the disputes between its own members, sometimes to admit ignorance, to divulge its staff's own anxiety and concerns, and to communicate uncertainty. Are the organizations prepared to undergo the ideological and administrative transformation we described in the public sphere of the 21st century?

### EID communication in the context of the public sphere

Organizations can try to contend with the gaps presented above or at least mitigate them in the public sphere through the use of risk communication. The term risk communication is used to describe the process of information dissemination and concomitant public reactions under conditions of uncertainty and threat. It is concerned not only with the nature of the risk itself, but also with the public's reactions to the risk messages, such as fears, concerns, and objections to the risk messages and the institutions and organizations that manage them. Risk communication judgments are, to some degree, a by-product of social, cultural, and psychological influences (Sandman, 2003; Slovic, 1999). The success of risk communication depends on the communicators' efforts to minimize the gap between the expert risk assessments and the public's perceptions, in order to create mutual feedback between the experts and the public (Fischhoff, 2004). Risk communication has many facets, one of which applies to crises, and is called "crisis communication."

Crisis communication is unique and distinct from communication in routine circumstances since in crisis situations the risk is not always familiar to the public and may not even be entirely familiar to the scientific community, so, action often needs to be taken before full information is available to the decision-makers. Furthermore, during crises there is constant change in the situation and thus improvisation and flexibility are essential, and officials have to be well trained and prepared for different scenarios (Edmunds, 2011; Reynolds, 2007; Reynolds and Seeger, 2012). In addition, due to the fact that many organizations and agencies are involved in this process, seamless coordination is essential in order to prevent redundancy, inefficiency, and interagency disagreements that can result in public confusion and anxiety (Reynolds and Seeger, 2012).

To better understand the public's feelings, needs and behaviors during crises and be attuned to its perceptions of risks, as well as its concerns and fears, the social system in which it operates must be understood (Cvetkovich and Lofstedt, 1999; Leiss, 1996).

The literature grants pride of place to crisis communication during epidemics. The importance of risk communication during epidemics is articulated in the following excerpt: "In the next influenza pandemic, be it now or in the future, be the virus mild or virulent, the single most important weapon against the disease will be a vaccine. The second most important will be communication" (Barry, 2009, p. 324). One of the specific forms of risk communication during an epidemic crisis is dubbed "Emerging Infectious Disease (EID) communication (Covello, 2003; Freimuth et al., 2000)." This approach draws on health promotion communication, crisis communication, and environmental/technological risk communication.

Emerging Infectious Disease encompasses a broad range of diseases (Holmes, 2008), covering previously unknown diseases (e.g. AIDS, Ebola), re-emerging diseases (e.g. tuberculosis, measles, pertussis), existing diseases that move to new places (e.g. West Nile virus, hepatitis), diseases that can no longer be controlled by once-effective drugs (e.g. malaria), and diseases exhibiting increased virulence (e.g. influenza in the 1918 epidemic). The emergence of these diseases is attributed to a number of factors, including the increasing growth and mobility of the world's population, overcrowding in cities with poor sanitation, unsanitary food preparation and overuse of antibiotics. Ecological changes are also believed to be a factor, for instance, those that lead to an increase in certain animal populations, which may in turn pave the way for the transfer of microbes to humans (Racaniello, 2004).

In books on risk communication, EID appears as part of a set of examples in the area of risk communication and public health (Bennett and Calman, 2008). Most of the risk communication books that appear as handbooks deal with a wide range of issues that are not limited to epidemics, such as environmental, safety, and health risks (Lundgren and McMakin, 2013). Most of the books discuss the planning, design, and evaluation of risk communication programs, including focusing on theoretical models in the area (Morgan et al., 2002; Witte et al.,2001). Some of the books on risk communication are devoted to characterizing crisis communication (Heath and O'Hair, 2010; Sellnow and Segger, 2013; Walaski, 2011).

Neither the books on crisis communication (Heath and O'Hair, 2010; Sellnow and Segger, 2013; Walaski, 2011) nor the articles about EID (Covello et al., 2001; Freimuth et al., 2000; Holmes, 2008) explain the difference between risk communication during epidemics, and risk communication during other crises and disasters such as earthquakes, nuclear reactor leaks, fires or bioterrorism. All ecological, health and security crises contain elements of uncertainty, unpredictability, and lack of control. Time is critical and magnifies the public's anxiety and concerns. In all cases, crisis knowledge management plays a central role. This means evaluating the public's risk perception throughout the crisis and providing the public with tools to deal with it, avoid it, and prevent it from getting worse. All cases involve a concomitant effort to manage public reaction: how the public perceives the risk, its anxiety and concerns, while addressing the public's cultural characteristics and maintaining ethical standards.

Yet, what distinguishes EID from other crises is the complexity of the "product." During an epidemic, the "product" being communicated is not just the epidemic itself, but also another element – the vaccine designed to prevent the disease. Therefore, organizations must deal with the uncertainty regarding the dynamic of the epidemic's spread and the ebbs and flows of its severity. This includes mortality, along with the uncertainty and the accompanying question of the vaccine's safety.

Organizations often focus on the vaccine in their crisis campaigns, but do not devote sufficient time and resources to communicating about the epidemic itself. The organizations are not always aware, as we noted in the Introduction, of the importance of the collective memory of epidemics, which influences the public's risk perception and ability to cope with the crisis.

Furthermore, the first condition for building effective communication is familiarity with the target audience's complex of needs and positions, or its social narrative. The narrative not only organizes information and events for people, but serves an instrument to infuse them with collective meaning (Bruner, 2002; Ricoeur, 1984). The collective narrative can also teach us about the collective subtext, which means the things that are not articulated explicitly and openly in the social context (Russell and Babrow, 2011). In reference to the risk narrative, Sandman's model (Sandman, 2003) and the mental models (Morgan et al., 2002) only stress the importance of knowing the audience's fears and concerns. The constructionist approach (Waddell, 1995) further stresses the need to know the target audience's system of beliefs, opinions, and fears, as well as those of the risk communicators and managers. The social constructivism approach believes that it is in fact the values, norms, and positions of the opinion leaders (the experts, the scientific community, the media) that influence the way they communicate and convey the message to the public, just as much as how the audience's norms and values influence the way it receives and is influenced by the transmission of the messages.

Although, organizations often state the importance of two-way communication, they are actually not reflective about their own tendencies and values in the way they communicate the risks. Understanding the social context where the epidemic occurs, along with understanding the collective memory of previous epidemics, serves not only to acquire and understand the common ground of the addressee – the public, as Billig (1996) noted, but also of the addresser, the policymakers.

Organizations are not the only ones that do not implement dialog with the public. As Holmes (2008) indicated, much of the EID communication literature deals with one-way transmission of facts to the public by experts. Little attention is paid to how differently various subpopulations conceptualize risk, or the idea that there is more to communication than the intentional transfer of information. Emerging infectious disease communication is often based on traditional health promotion or emergency/crisis communication literature, where it is assumed that the only "enemy" is the disease, that the right course of action is obvious, and that the expertise (coming from a public health establishment and assumed to be value-free) will not be questioned. Research tends to be limited to exploring barriers to understanding or to education, in order to facilitate better message development.

## *From linear to complex and a constantly changing framework*

The risk communication aspect of pandemic outbreaks has developed to such an extent, that it threatens to almost overshadow the pure healthcare aspect of virus containment. To cope with epidemic crises, there have been advances in theories and models of risk communication and crisis communication, and specifically in EID communication. Some of these theories and models draw heavily from crisis management theories such as the Three-Stage Model (Ray, 1999) and Fink's Four-Stage Cycle (Fink, 1986). Yet, these models are overly general and tend to be structured in linear, hierarchic terms that downplay the environmental-cultural aspect of the public. Few models of crisis management have attempted to address the environmental and cultural aspects of crises, such as Turner's Six-Stage Sequence of Failure in Foresight (Turner, 1976), which emphasizes social processes that help constitute order, including the development of social norms, processes, and practices. Turner's work conceptualizes crisis as a "cultural collapse," where the normative and social structure is no longer "accurate or adequate" (Turner, 1976).

The organizations' understanding that coping with an epidemic crisis should occur by situating the public sociologically and psychologically has led to changes regarding the role of communication in crisis management. There has been much progress since the predominance of the principle of the "hypodermic needle," where the public is "injected" with the message. For example, the CDC's CERC model has given pride of place to feedback and two-way communication between the organization and the public (Courtney et al., 2003). Another notable model is the Four-Channel Model that focuses on transactive communication, situating the public at the center and viewing it as an active partner and not merely a recipient (Pechta et al., 2010). This repositioning of the public as an active participant is facilitated by new mobile technologies, especially smartphones and internet-based tools.

Although the consensus is that this theory is updated and relevant, in practice, the information flow remains unilateral in many countries. The call for "engagement" of the public is a concept that still reflects a passive audience to be engaged, and does not take into account the polyvocality of the public and a reality in which the opinions and knowledge of the public "compete" with those of the health authorities. Moreover, the understanding that the public in the 21st century is a full partner necessitates a greater understanding of the social and technological realms in which the public operates.

In order to deal with the paradox faced by organizations in the public sphere, we conceptualized our approach through a framework formulated in the TELL ME FP7 Project (Gesser-Edelsburg et al., 2015). Unlike models such as those mentioned above, this framework is not predicated on arrows connecting the organizations and the public, but rather, refocuses in greater detail on the "behind-the-scenes" of the public sphere. The proposed framework is not based on a hierarchical, linear structure. Nor is it an attempt to shape or funnel reality into clear, linear spreadsheets, as some guidelines do

(Reynolds, 2007). For this reason, rather then using arrows, the diagram describing the proposed framework (see Figure 1.1) is constructed as a response to the reality of outbreak communication. The structure of the framework is complex, which corresponds to a complex and constantly-changing reality. It draws inspiration from the rhizome theory proposed by the philosophers Deleuze and Guattari, which suggests an alternative to linear models based on binaries, and emphasizes multiple connections and heterogeneity. Also like the rhizome, this model is *not* based on hierarchical relations, but on relations that proliferate in many directions, and emphasize many possible connections. One principle of the rhizome is the "principle of signifying rupture" (Bogue, 1989), which states that ruptures or obstacles do not cause a breakdown, but instead any sort of disruption leads to a new, productive flow of movement. The TELL ME project aimed to map a reality in which communication is multi-directional, proliferating in many directions, and in which the average citizen plays an active role in the communication process. All the components of our model encompass

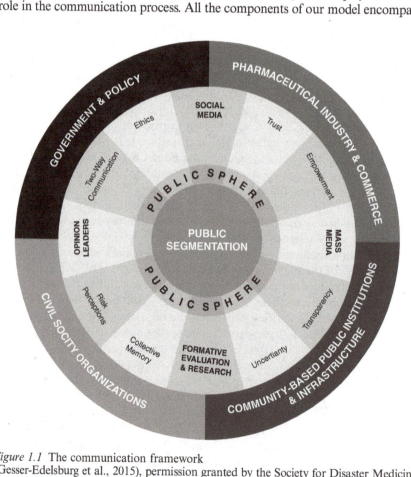

*Figure 1.1* The communication framework
(Gesser-Edelsburg et al., 2015), permission granted by the Society for Disaster Medicine and Public Health.

the public sphere. We present the framework diagram in order to illustrate that the public sphere is positioned at the center, deemphasizing boundaries between it and seven key components (such as opinion leaders, formal stakeholders, the media, etc.) that encompass and embody it (see Figure 1.1).

This framework shows that different elements overlap, an overlap which reflects the fact that communication does not have clear-cut limits. Formal stakeholders are not at the center of this model, but rather encompass (and form part of) the public. This is where concepts like transparency, risk perception, collective memory, trust, and ethics come into play. Figure 1.1 illustrates the transformation of the public from recipient to equal partner. It demonstrates the elimination of the hierarchy between the organization and the public, and at the same time indicates that the solution to the organizations' paradox can be illustrated in the way the organizations embrace the public sphere, metaphorically surrounding its collective memory and maintaining its boundaries, without attempting to dictate to the public unilaterally. In this depiction, stakeholders have a constant presence in the public sphere, not only during times of crisis.

## References

Achenbach, J., Dennis, B., and Hogan, C. (2014). American doctor infected with Ebola returns to U.S. *The Washington Post*, August 2. Available at: www.washingtonpost.com/national/health-science/us-confirms-2-americans-with-ebola-coming-home-for-treatment/2014/08/01/c20a27cc-1995-11e4-9e3b-7f2f110c6265_story.html

Adler, R. E. (2004). *Medical Firsts: From Hippocrates to the Human Genome*. Hoboken, NJ: John Wiley & Sons, Inc.

Alexander, M. (2003). *Calling the Shots: Childhood Vaccination – One Family's Journey*. London: Jessica Kingsley Publishers.

Barry, J. M. (2009). Pandemics: avoiding the mistakes of 1918. *Nature*, 459(7245), 324–325.

Bartlett, S. J. (2005). *The Pathology of Man: A Study of Human Evil*. Springfield, IL: Charles C. Thomas Publisher.

Baxby, D. (1984). A death from inoculated smallpox in the English Royal Family. *Medical History*, 28(03), 303–307.

Bennett, P., and Calman, K. (2008). *Risk Communication and Public Health*. Oxford: Oxford Medical Publications.

Bergen, T. (2014). Worst disease outbreaks in history. Available at: www.msn.com/en-us/health/medical/worst-disease-outbreaks-in-history/ss-BBaE52y#image=8

Billig, M. (1996). *Arguing and Thinking: A Rhetorical Approach to Social Psychology*. Cambridge: Cambridge University Press.

Boccaccio, G. (1973). *The Decameron of Giovanni Boccaccio* (trans. R. Aldington). New York: Dell Laurel Books.

Bogue, R. (1989). *Deleuze and Guattari*. London: Routledge.

Bonanni, P., and Santos, J. I. (2011). Vaccine evolution. *Perspectives in Vaccinology*, 1(1), 1–24.

Branato, K. (2015). History's deadliest epidemics. Available at: www.cnbc.com/2014/10/17/historys-deadliest-epidemics.html

Brennan, B., and Hall, W. (2009). Putting planning into practice: the communications response to H1N1. A Global Communications Conference sponsored by the Pan American Health Organization and the United States Department of Health and Human Services, Washington, DC, 22 July.

Bristow, N. K. (2012). *American Pandemic: The Lost Worlds of the 1918 Influenza Epidemic*. Oxford: Oxford University Press.

Bruner, J. S. (2002). *Making Stories: Law, Literature, Life*. New York: Farrar, Straus and Giroux.

Byrne, J. P. (2006). *Daily Life during the Black Death*. Westport, CT: Greenwood Press.

Case, C. L., and Chung, K. T. (1997). Montagu and Jenner: The campaign against smallpox. *SIM News*, 47(2), 58–60.

Cassoobhoy, A. (2014). CDC: Ebola questions and answers. *WebMD*, August 8. Available at: www.webmd.com/news/20140808/ebola-questions-answers

Christian, H. (2011). Plague and persecution: The Black Death and early modern witch hunts. Available at: http://aladinrc.wrlc.org/bitstream/handle/1961/9878/Christian%2c%20Helen%20-%20Spring%20%2711.pdf?sequence=1

Cohn, J. S. K. (2002). The black death: End of a paradigm. *The American Historical Review*, 107(3), 703–738.

CohnJr, S. K. (2010). *Cultures of Plague: Medical Thinking at the End of the Renaissance*. Oxford: Oxford University Press. Courtney, J., Cole, G., and Reynolds, B. (2003). How the CDC is meeting the training demands of emergency risk communication. *Journal of Health Communication*, 8(suppl. 1), 128–129.

Covello, V. T. (2003). Best practices in public health risk and crisis communication. *Journal of Health Communication*, 8(S1), 5–8, 148–151.

Covello, V. T., Peters, R. G., Wojtecki, J. G., and Hyde, R. C. (2001). Risk communication, the West Nile virus epidemic, and bioterrorism: Responding to the communication challenges posed by the intentional or unintentional release of a pathogen in an urban setting. *Journal of Urban Health : Bulletin of the New York Academy of Medicine*, 78(2), 382–391.

Cunningham, A. (2008). Epidemics, pandemics, and the Doomsday Scenario. *Historically Speaking*, 9(7), 29–31.

Cvetkovich, G., and Lofsted, R. E. (1999). *Social Trust and the Management of Risk*. London: Earthscan Publications.

Daintith, J. (2008). *Biographical Encyclopedia of Scientists*. Boca Raton, FL: CRC Press.

De Paolo, C. (2006). *Epidemic Disease and Human Understanding: A Historical Analysis of Scientific and Other Writings*. Jefferson, NC: McFarland and Company.

Dolber, C. (2010). Containing contagion: Perception and prevention of plague in the late Middle Ages. Available at: www.academia.edu/4796647/Containing_Contagion_Perception_and_Prevention_of_Plague_in_the_Late_Middle_Ages

Dominus, S. (2009). In 1918 flu outbreak, a cool head prevailed. *The New York Times*, April 30. Available at: www.nytimes.com/2009/05/01/nyregion/01bigcity.html?_r=2

Driedger, S. M., Cooper, E., Jardine, C., Furgal, C., and Bartlett, J. (2013). Communicating risk to Aboriginal peoples: First nations and metis responses to H1N1 risk messages. *PLOS One*, 8(8), e71106.

Durbach, N. (2000). 'They might as well brand us': Working-class resistance to compulsory vaccination in Victorian England. *Social History of Medicine*, 13(1), 45–63.

Dutta, M. J. (2007). Communicating about culture and health: theorizing culture-centered and cultural sensitivity approaches. *Communication Theory*, 17(3), 304–328.

Edmunds, M. (2011). Risk communications for public health preparedness. Available at: http://trams.jhsph.edu/trams/views/content/fileLibrary/tID217/cphp_edmunds_full.pdf (accessed April 21, 2016).

Fenner, F., Henderson, D. A., Arita, I., Jezek, Z., and Ladnyi, I. D. (1988). *Smallpox and Its Eradication*. Geneva: World Health Organization.

Fernandez, M., and Philipps, D. (2014). Death of Thomas Eric Duncan in Dallas fuels alarm over Ebola . *The New York Times*, October 8. Available at: www.nytimes.com/2014/10/09/us/ebola-us-thomas-eric-duncan.html?_r=0

Fink, S. (1986). *Crises Management: Planning for the Inevitable*. New York: American Management Association.

Fischhoff, B. (2004). A diagnostic for risk communication failers. In W. Leiss and D. Powell (Eds.), *Mad Cows and Mother's Milk: The Perils of Poor Risk Communication* (2nd edition, pp. 26–40). Montreal: McGill-Queen's University Press.

Fischhoff, B. (2005). Scientifically sound pandemic risk communication. Paper presented at the U.S. House Science Committee Briefing: Gaps in the National Flu Preparedness Plan, Social Science Planning and Response, December 14.

Foa, A. (2000). *The Jews of Europe after the Black Death* (trans. A. Grover). Berkeley, CA: University of California Press.

Freemon, F. R. (2005). Bubonic plague in the Book of Samuel. *Journal of the Royal Society of Medicine*, 98(9), 436.

Freimuth, V., Linnan, H. W., and Potter, P. (2000). Communicating the threat of emerging infections to the public. *Emerging Infectious Diseases*, 6(4), 337–347.

Frewer, L., Hunt, S., Brennan, M., Kuznesof, S., Ness, M., and Ritson, C. (2003). The views of scientific experts on how the public conceptualize uncertainty. *Journal of Risk Research*, 6(1), 75–85.

Furgal, C., Powell, S., and Myers, H. (2005). Digesting the message about contaminants and country foods in the Canadian north: A review and recommendations for future research and action. *Arctic*, 58(2), 103–114.

Gesser-Edelsburg, A., Mordini, E., James, J. J., Greco, D., and Green, M. S. (2014). Risk communication recommendations and implementation during emerging infectious diseases: A case study of the 2009 H1N1 influenza pandemic. *Disaster Medicine and Public Health Preparedness*, 8(2), 158–169.

Gesser-Edelsburg, A., Shir-Raz, Y., Walter, N., Mordini, E., Dimitriou, D., James, J. J., et al. (2015). The public sphere in emerging infectious disease communication: Recipient or active and vocal partner? *Disaster Medicine and Public Health Preparedness*, 9(4), 447–458.

Gray, L., MacDonald, C., Mackie, B., Paton, D., Johnston, D., and Baker, M. G. (2012). Community responses to communication campaigns for influenza A (H1N1): a focus group study. *BMC Public Health*, 12, 205.

Grey, D. J. R. (2016). "To bring this useful invention into fashion in England": Mary Wortley Montagu as medical expert. In T. Barnard (Ed.), *British Women and the Intellectual World in the Long Eighteenth Century*. New York: Routledge. pp. 15–32.

Griffin, J. P. (2000). Bubonic plague in biblical times. *Journal of the Royal Society of Medicine*, 93(8), 449.

Gross, C. P., and Sepkowitz, K. A. (1998). The myth of the medical breakthrough: Smallpox, vaccination, and Jenner reconsidered. *International Journal of Infectious Diseases*, 3(1), 54–60.

Guerrini, A. (2003). *Experimenting with Humans and Animals: From Galen to Animal Rights*. Baltimore, MD: The Johns Hopkins University Press.

Habermas, J. (1989). *The Structural Transformation of the Public Sphere: An Inquiry into a Category of Bourgeois Society*. Cambridge: Polity Press.

Habermas, J. (2004). *The Divided West*. Malden, MA: Polity Press.

Härtl, G. (2013). Novel coronavirus: The challenge of communicating about a virus which one knows little about. *Eastern Mediterranean Health Journal*, 19(suppl. 1), S26–S30.

Health Canada. (2005). Information: Canada's national and international collaboration on pandemic influenza planning. Available at: https://flutrackers.com/forum/forum/canada/h5n1-tracking-ag/30578-canada-pandemic-preparedness-documentation (accessed July 10, 2008).

Heath, R. L., and O'Hair, H. D. (2010). *Handbook of Risk and Crisis Communication*. New York: Routledge.

Henderson, D. A. (2009). *Smallpox: The Death of a Disease – The Inside Story of Eradicating a Worldwide Killer*. Amherst, NY: Prometheus Books.

Holmes, B. J. (2008). Communicating about emerging infectious disease: The importance of research. *Health, Risk and Society*, 10(4), 349–360.

Horgan, J. (2014). Justinian's plague. Available at: www.ancient.eu/article/782/

Jankowski, N., and Van Selm, M. (2000). The promise and practice of public debate in cyberspace. In K. L. Hacker and J. van Dijk (Eds.), *Digital Democracy: Issues of Theory and Practice* (pp. 149–165). London: Sage.

Krimsky, S., and Plough, A. (1988). *Environmental Hazards: Communicating Risks as a Social Process*. Dover, MA: Auburn House Publishing Company.

Lam, P. P., and McGreen, A. (2011). Communication strategies for the 2009 Influenza A (H1N1) pandemic. Available at: http://nccid.ca/publications/communication-strategies-for-the-2009-influenza-a-h1n1-pandemic/ (accessed April 20, 2016).

Leiss, W. (1996). Three phases in the evolution of risk communication practice. *Annals AAPSS*, 545, 85–94.

Leung, A. K. C. (1996). "Variolation" and vaccination in late imperial China, ca 1570–1911. In S. A. Plotkin (Ed.), *History of Vaccine Development* (pp. 5–12). New York: Springer.

Levack, B. P. (1995). *The Witch-Hunt in Early Modern Europe* (3rd edition). New York: Routledge.

Levy, R. S. (2005). *Antisemitism: A Historical Encyclopedia of Prejudice and Persecution* (Vol. 1). Santa Barbara, CA: ABC-CLIO, Inc.

Lindell, M. K., and Perry, R. W. (2004). *Communicating Environmental Risk in Multiethnic Communities*. Thousand Oaks, CA: Sage.

Lundgren, R. E., and McMakin, A. H. (2013). *Risk Communication: A Handbook for Communicating Environmental, Safety, and Health Risks* (5th edition). Piscataway, NJ: IEEE Press.

MacKenzie, D., and Marshall, M. (2009). Timeline: The secret history of swine flu. *New Scientist*, October 29. Available at: www.newscientist.com/article/dn18063-timeline-the-secret-history-of-swine-flu/ (accessed April 22, 2016).

Mackowiak, P. A., and Sehdev, P. S. (2002). The origin of quarantine. *Clinical Infectious Diseases*, 35(9), 1071–1072.

Massey, P. D., Miller, A., Saggers, S., Durrheim, D. N., Speare, R., Taylor, K., *et al.* (2011). Australian Aboriginal and Torres Strait Islander communities and the development of pandemic influenza containment strategies: community voices and community control. *Health Policy*, 103(2–3), 184–190.

Massey, P. D., Pearce, G., Taylor, K. A., Orcher, L., Saggers, S., and Durrheim, D. N. (2009). Reducing the risk of pandemic influenza in Aboriginal communities. *Rural Remote Health*, 9(3), 1290.

Matovinovic, J. (1969). A short history of quarantine (Victor C. Vaughan). *University of Michigan Medical Center Journal*, 35(4), 224–228.

Maurice, J. (2015). Measles outbreak in DR Congo an "epidemic emergency." *The Lancet*, 386(9997), 943.

Ministry of Health Republic of Botswana. (2014). Ebola virus alert. Available at: www. moh.gov.bw/ebola.html (accessed Sept. 11, 2014).

Mitchell, P. (2012). *Contagious Metaphor*. London: Bloomsbury Academic.

Moore, J. (n.d.) Deadly diseases: Epidemics throughout history. Available at: http:// edition.cnn.com/interactive/2014/10/health/epidemics-through-history/

Moore, R. I. (2007). *The Formation of a Persecuting Society: Authority Deviance in Western Europe, 950–1250* (2nd edition). Oxford: Blackwell Publishing.

Morgan, M. G., Fischhoff, B., Bostrom, A., and Atman, C. J. (2002). *Risk Communication: A Mental Models Approach*. New York: Cambridge University Press.

National Geographic Staff. (2014). Graphic: as Ebola's death toll rises, Remembering history's worst epidemics. *National Geographic*, October 25, vol. 2015.

National Health Service. (2005). Pandemic flu: UK influenza pandemic contingency plan. Available at: http://webarchive.nationalarchives.gov.uk/20130107105354/http://www. dh.gov.uk/prod_consum_dh/groups/dh_digitalassets/@dh/@en/documents/digitalasset/ dh_4121744.pdf

Needham, J. (1980). *China and the Origins of Immunology*. Hong Kong: Centre of Asian Studies, University of Hong Kong.

NHS. (2016). The history of vaccination. Available at: www.nhs.uk/conditions/vaccina tions/pages/the-history-of-vaccination.aspx?tabname=Children%20and%20teens

NIH. (2013). Smallpox: A great and terrible scourge (variolation). Available at: www. nlm.nih.gov/exhibition/smallpox/sp_variolation.html

Nirenberg, D. (1996). *Communities of Violence: Persecution of Minorities in the Middle Ages* Princeton, NJ: Princeton University Press.

Nutton, V. (1990). The reception of Fracastoro's theory of contagion: The seed that fell among thorns? *Osiris*, 6, 196–234.

Oosterwijk, S. (2009). 'Fro Paris to Inglond'? The 'Danse macabre' in Text and Image in Late-Medieval England. Doctoral thesis, Leiden University. Available at: https:// openaccess.leidenuniv.nl/handle/1887/13873

Oosterwijk, S. (2012). *Dance of Death*. Oxford: Oxford Bibliographies.

Pappas, G., Seitaridis, S., Akritidis, N., and Tsianos, E. (2003). Infectious diseases in cinema: Virus hunters and killer microbes. *Clinical Infectious Diseases: An Official Publication of the Infectious Diseases Society of America*, 37(7), 939–942.

Pechta, L. E., Brandenburg, D. C., and Seeger, M. W. (2010). Understanding the dynamics of emergency communication: Propositions for a four-channel model. *Journal of Homeland Security and Emergency Management*, 7(1), 1–18.

Racaniello, V. R. (2004). Emerging infectious diseases. *The Journal of Clinical Investigation*, 113(6), 796–798.

Ray, S. J. (1999). *Strategic Communication in Crisis Management: Lessons from the Airline Industry*. Westport, CT: Quorum Books.

Razzell, P. E. (1977). *The Conquest of Smallpox: The Impact of Inoculation on Smallpox Mortality in Eighteenth Century Britain*. London: Caliban Books.

Reynolds, B. (2007). Crisis and emergency risk communication: pandemic influenza. Available at: www.bt.cdc.gov/cerc/resources/pdf/cerc-pandemicflu-oct07.pdf

Reynolds, B., and Seeger, M. (2012). *Crisis and Emergency Risk Communication.* Atlanta, GA: Centers for Disease Control and Prevention.

Ricoeur, P. (1984). *Time and Narrative.* (Vol. 1) (trans. K. McLaughlin and D. Pellauer). Chicago: University of Chicago Press.

Riedel, S. (2005). Edward Jenner and the history of smallpox and vaccination. *Proceedings (Baylor University Medical Center)*, 18(1), 21–25.

Rosenberg, C. E. (2008). Siting epidemic disease: 3 centuries of American history. *The Journal of Infectious Diseases*, 197 (suppl. 1), S4–6.

Rudge, S., and Massey, P. D. (2010). Responding to pandemic (H1N1) 2009 influenza in Aboriginal communities in NSW through collaboration between NSW Health and the Aboriginal community-controlled health sector. *NSW Public Health Bulletin*, 21(1–2), 26–29.

Russell, L. D., and Babrow, A. S. (2011). Risk in the making: Narrative, problematic integration, and the social construction of risk. *Communication Theory*, 21(3), 239–260.

Sandman, P. (1989). Hazard versus outrage in the public perception of risk. In V. T. Covello, D. B. McCallum and M. T. Pavlova (Eds.), *Effective Risk Communication: The Role and Responsibility of Government and Nongovernment Organizations* (pp. 45–49). New York: Plenum Press.

Sandman, P. (2003). Four kinds of risk communication. *The Synergist*, 8, 26–27.

Sandman, P. (2007). Understanding the risk: What frightens rarely kills. *Nieman Reports*, Spring, 59–66.

Sellnow, T. L., and Segger, M. W. (2013). *Theorizing Crisis Communication.* Malden, MA: Wiley-Blackwell.

Shurkin, J. N. (1979). *The Invisible Fire: The Story of Mankind's Victory over the Ancient Scourge of Smallpox.* New York: Putnam.

Slovic, P. (1999). Trust, emotion, sex, politics, and science: Surveying the risk-assessment battlefield. *Risk Analysis*, 19(4), 689–701.

Slovic, P. (2000). *The Perception of Risk.* London: Earthscan.

Stuard, S. M. (1992). *A State of Deference: Ragusa/Dubrovnik in the Medieval Centuries.* Philadelphia, PA: University of Pennsylvania Press.

Thackeray, R., Neiger, B. L., Burton, S. H., and Thackeray, C. R. (2013). Analysis of the purpose of state health departments' tweets: Information sharing, engagement, and action. *Journal of Medical Internet Research*, 15(11), e255.

Turner, B. M. (1976). The organizational and inter-organizational development of disasters. *Administrative Science Quarterly*, 21(3), 378–397.

Van De Donk, W., Loader, B. D., Nixon, P. G., and Rucht, D. (2004). *Cyberprotest: New Media, Citizens and Social Movements.* London: Routledge.

Van Os, R., Jankowski, N. W., and Vergeer, M. (2007). Political communication about Europe on the Internet during the 2004 European Parliament election campaign in nine EU member states. *European Societies*, 9(5), 755–775.

Velimirovic, B., and Velimirovic, H. (1989). Plague in Vienna. *Review of Infectious Diseases*, 11(5), 808–826.

Vidal, P., Tibayrenc, M., and Gonzalez, J. P. (2007). Infectious disease and arts. In M. Tibayrenc (Ed.), *Encyclopedia of Infectious Diseases: Modern Methodologies.* Hoboken, NJ: John Wiley & Sons, Inc.

Waddell, C. (1995). Defining sustainable development: a case study in environmental communication. *Technical Communication Quarterly*, 4(2), 201–216.

Walaski, P. M. (2011). *Risk and Crisis Communications: Methods and Messages.* Hoboken, NJ: John Wiley & Sons, Inc.

Wallis, F. (2010). *Medieval Medicine: A Reader* (Vol. 15). Toronto, Ontario: University of Toronto Press Incorporated.

WHO. (2005). WHO outbreak communication guidelines. Available at: www.who.int/csr/resources/publications/WHO_CDS_2005_28en.pdf

WHO. (2008a). *International Health Regulations* (2nd edition). Available at: http://whqlibdoc.who.int/publications/2008/9789241580410_eng.pdf

WHO. (2008b). *World Health Organization Outbreak Communication Planning Guide.* Available at: www.who.int/ihr/elibrary/WHOOutbreakCommsPlanngGuide.pdf (accessed October 20, 2012).

WHO. (2014). *Ebola Virus Disease in Guinea: Disease Outbreak News.* Geneva: World Health Organization.

WHO. (2015). HIV/AIDS: Fact sheet N°360. Available at: www.who.int/mediacentre/factsheets/fs360/en/

Williams, G. (2010). *Angel of Death: The Story of Smallpox.* New York: Palgrave Macmillan.

Witte, K., Meyer, G., and Martell, D. (2001). *Effective Health Risk Messages: A Step-By-Step Guide.* Thousand Oaks, CA: Sage.

Zahler, D. (2009). *The Black Death.* Minneapolis, MN: Twenty-First Century Books.

# 2 The Challenge of Digital Media for Health Organizations

As the plague in Oran slowly spreads, Dr. Rieux, Albert Camus's protagonist in *The Plague*, tries to convince the town authorities to take action and declare an epidemic. Unfortunately, the officials are slow to react. Dr. Richard, the chairman of the Oran Medical Association, argues that "it was a mistake to paint too gloomy a picture, and, moreover, the disease hadn't been proved to be contagious." The officials, afraid to arouse public alarm, refuse even to officially admit that plague had broken out. Instead, they refer to it as a "special type of fever." Camus's description of the authorities' reaction to the plague was not detached from reality. In 1576, in the midst of the plague that struck northern Italy, the Bishop of Verona criticized the government's "refusal to use the 'formidable name' of the plague," as one of the major factors that led to chaos and uprisings in the city (Cohn Jr, 2010, p. 264).

Today, as Samarajiva and Gunawardene (2013) argue, the controlled dissemination of information is no longer an option for any government or health authority. This major challenge is demonstrated in almost every outbreak in recent years, beginning with the 2002–2003 SARS outbreak. The SARS (Severe Acute Respiratory Syndrome), which eventually infected 8,096 people in 27 countries and killed 774, broke out in November 2002 (WHO, 2003a) in the southern Chinese province of Guangdong (WHO, 2003b). Yet, three months later, the Chinese government was still trying to contain information about it and actively suppressed news of the outbreak (Yu and Madoff, 2004).

Nevertheless, a post written by a Chinese citizen managed to permeate the Chinese wall of secrecy. In his post, "Ben" described an illness that began like a cold, but killed people in days (Drexler, 2008). On February 9, 2003, Catherine Strommen, a teacher from California, read the post on Teachers.net, an international online community for teachers, and emailed it to a friend, Dr. Stephan Cunnion, a consultant in the field of infectious diseases and a retired Navy physician. After failing to find any information on the Web about this strange outbreak, Dr. Cunnion posted an email to ProMED-mail (Drexler, 2008), an electronic mailing list run by the International Society for Infectious Diseases, which alerts subscribers to the spread of infectious diseases and toxins (Cunnion, 2003):

Date: 10 Feb 2003

This morning I received this e-mail and then searched your archives and found nothing that pertained to it. Does anyone know anything about this problem?

Have you heard of an epidemic in Guangzhou? An acquaintance of mine from a teacher's chat room lives there and reports that the hospitals there have been closed and people are dying.

Stephen O. Cunnion, MD, PhD,

MPH International Consultants in Health, Inc

Member ASTM&H, ISTM

Ben's report quickly spread by email to tens of thousands of Americans, enabling the world to learn about the fatal outbreak. That same day, the WHO sent a query to Beijing, asking for information about the outbreak, and on February 11, the Chinese Ministry of Health officially reported to the WHO that an acute respiratory syndrome had infected 305 people and caused five deaths (Brookes and Khan, 2005).

Other examples, including the most recent ones, such as the 2014 Ebola epidemic, the 2015 measles outbreak in California and the Zika outbreak in 2016, further illustrate that in the age of social media, when the authorities hesitate or are reluctant to declare an outbreak, the first indication of it comes from the public.

On July 24, 2014, four days after the first case of the Ebola virus in Nigeria (WHO, 2014), Twitter users were talking about the case, discussing the disease trends, as well as its risk factors and prevention measures. Among the messages tweeted were: "#EbolaVirus 1st case discovered Lagos, pls spread the word"; and "Guys, #EbolaVirus is in Lagos. Be informed. Be careful." The tweets, reaching 1,196,793 people on the first day alone, started to circulate 3–7 days prior to the official announcement about the first suspected patient (Odlum and Yoon, 2015). Similarly, in the 2015 measles outbreak in California, the story broke by way of a post tweeted by a pediatrician from San Diego, who wrote about the cases diagnosed and their connection to the Disney parks. The formal statement by the California Department of Public Health was only issued on January 7– over 15 hours later (Matthews, 2015).

## The public's role in knowledge generation and dissemination

Many studies have indicated that in emergency situations, the public seeks information in order to reduce uncertainty, and will use whatever means available to obtain it (Boyle et al., 2004; Hughes et al. 2008; Mileti and Darlington, 1997; Stiegler et al., 2011). In the event of an epidemic, people want to know the risk of infection, how sick they could become if infected, and what can be done to prevent and treat the disease. To be able to make decisions about using vaccines and drugs, they need information that will enable them to assess the risks and benefits involved in it (Henrich and Holmes, 2011). Over the last decade, social media have become a primary source of information. Even while still in their infancy, social networking sites were awash with information and messages pertaining to the 2009 H1N1 outbreak. Twitter messages containing the term "swine flu" rose from almost zero to 125,000 per day by May 1, 2009 (Petrie and Faasse, 2009). According to Nielsenwire, in some accounts there were 10,000 tweets that mentioned "swine flu" over the course of an hour (Davies, 2009). Blogs showed a similar pattern, with a large increase in the percentage of blogs mentioning "swine flu." Additionally, at the height of the outbreak, there were more than 500 Facebook groups dedicated to H1N1 discussions (Petrie and Faasse, 2009).

Likewise, several studies have shown that during the 2011 H7N9 flu pandemic in China, social networking activity increased (Fung et al., 2013; Gu et al., 2014; Zhang et al., 2015; Zhang and Gao, 2014).

Regarding the Ebola epidemic, the first case on U.S. soil was followed by a rapid increase in online activity mentioning Ebola on Twitter and Google (Fung et al., 2014). Within 24 hours, there was an 11-fold increase in Ebola-related tweets across the USA (Rodriguez-Morales et al.,2015). Similarly, as soon as the first known case of Zika in the United States was reported in Texas in 2016, the virus became a trending topic on various social media platforms, including Facebook, Twitter and mobile apps. Zika has been linked to a rise in severe birth defects in Brazil. In addition, the first U.S. case was followed by an increase in Google searches for Zika, with the Texas cities of Garland, Dallas and Grapevine topping the list (Reuters, 2016).

Moreover, studies have consistently shown that the public not only seeks information during epidemics, but, rather, takes an active role in generating knowledge, including information filtering, interpretation, amplification, and dissemination (Chew and Eysenbach, 2010). For example, Chew and Eysenbach (2010) found that during the 2009 H1N1 outbreak, Twitter was used primarily to disseminate information, as the most common type of content shared (52.6%) was resource-related posts. Similarly, during the 2011 H7N9 flu pandemic, social media were used as a platform to share information and for collaboration among different users (Zhang and Gao, 2014). Furthermore, it was found that social media were significantly faster in reporting new cases than conventional reporting sites (Zhang et al., 2015), and that the information disseminated through social media originated from credible sources (Chew and Eysenbach, 2010). Only 4.5% of the tweets analyzed by Chew and Eysenbach (2010) during the 2009 H1N1 outbreak were categorized as containing misinformation.

## The digital media: sharing personal experiences, opinions and concerns

Social media, forums and blogs have become more than just an important tool for disseminating, sharing and seeking health information during epidemics. They also serve as a medium for expressing anxiety and concerns about illnesses (Petrie and Faasse, 2009; Tausczik et al., 2012); sharing personal experiences and opinions (Chew and Eysenbach, 2010); and discussing treatments and prevention measures during outbreaks (Bults et al., 2011; Signorini et al.,

2011). For instance, in Chew and Eysenbach's (2010) study, the second most frequent content shared during the 2009 H1N1 outbreak (22.5%) was personal experiences, followed by humor (12.7%), concern (11.7%), and questions (10.3%). In Israel, two days after the Health Ministry announced the discontinuation of use and market recall of all Sci-b-vac vaccines – Hepatitis B vaccines given routinely in Israel to babies 0–6 months old (State of Israel Ministry of Health, 2015a), parents whose children had received the vaccine were discussing their concerns about potential risks on forums and on Facebook (Asulin-Karutchi, 2015; Rotem, 2015). The Health Ministry's announcement stressed it was merely a precautionary recall, "due to a technical flaw in packaging." Yet, many worried parents felt this explanation was vague and unclear. Some of them turned to the Web for additional information, found the recall announcement released by the company abroad, which was more detailed, and published it online, along with criticism of the Ministry of Health:

> When a recall for cars is announced due to problems with the brakes – we all understand the danger and rush to the garage ... But when the public reads that there is a vaccine recall – what should parents whose babies received this manufacturer's vaccine do? Here is the announcement from abroad about the same Hepatitis vaccine ... Read it and take a screenshot of the link before it disappears/is deleted.
>
> (Rotem, 2015)

Following these discussions, the next day, August 2, the Ministry of Health published a clarification, expanding on the explanation for the recall: "In sample testing performed as part of the vaccine's routine manufacturing and packaging process at the factory, a suspicion arose that tiny cracks were forming in the vaccine ampules" (State of Israel Ministry of Health, 2015b).

The issue of vaccination is one of the major sources of concern raised in social media. For example, during the 2009 H1N1 outbreak, there was a pronounced rise in use of social media to express concerns related to vaccine side effects or to vaccination risks (Signorini et al., 2011). Furthermore, those who refused to vaccinate reported more information-seeking behavior, and solicited advice more frequently on their social network than those who had vaccinated (Bults et al., 2011). This discourse of doubts and concerns, as well as the anti-vaccination messages, may influence some people's vaccination decisions and increase vaccination hesitancy and refusal trends among parents, which have been on the rise in recent years (Betsch et al., 2010; Kata, 2012).

## The authorities' increasing use of the social media

Over the past decade, leading international health authorities, health ministries, and local governments have invested financial and human resources in order to mitigate the gaps in social media that were conspicuous in previous health crises between the authorities and the public, and offer greater presence in social media. The World Health Organization now has Facebook and Twitter accounts, as do the Centers for Disease Control and Prevention (CDC) and numerous health-related schools and departments, scientists, and health-focused news outlets. CDC has developed an online toolkit to aid public health practitioners disseminate information and foster partnerships with consumers through the social media. Despite numerous barriers that often hinder the adoption of new technology in government organizations, studies indicate a majority of state health departments (60%–82%) use at least one social media application (Harris et al., 2013).

The 2009 H1N1 influenza pandemic was the WHO's first experience with social media. The organization used Twitter to update the daily rise in cases of infection, and also monitored what was being said about the WHO in the social media. However, without any clear policy or experience with dealing with this new public sphere, its engagement was limited at that time (Härtl, 2013). By examining tweets sent during the outbreak, health authorities were able to identify and respond promptly to public concerns. Similarly, following natural disasters such as earthquakes and wildfires, social media have been used by emergency response organizations for monitoring and responding (Wong et al., 2015).

Along with the international organizations, health organizations at the national level also began to take advantage of social media during the 2009 outbreak. For example, tweets made by the Virginia Health Department about the location of vaccination sites led people to flock there within minutes (Merchant et al., 2011). Since 2009, the organizations have progressed in using social media in the following categories: (1) Using social networks and greater interaction with the public; (2) Increased use of surveillance tools in programs in order to locate discourse in the social media. In what follows, we will offer details regarding each of these categories.

### *Using social networks for education and distributing information*

The use of social media by public health organizations helps reach people when and where it is most convenient for them to receive health information. This type of communication can be integrated into health communication strategies to improve, reach, and promote campaign messages and organization activities (Bergeron et al., 2013).

Today, government agencies are increasingly interested in interacting with the populations they serve. State public health departments markedly expanded their use of social media from 2011 to 2014, viewing it as an effective, low-cost means to reach their audiences. Furthermore, new guidelines entitled "Digital Governmental Strategy" outline specific steps for governmental agencies to make digital information more "customer-centric" (Herman, 2013).

The National Public Health Information Coalition (NPHIC) reported that 82% of state health agencies use both Facebook and Twitter, versus 44% in

August 2011. "This illustrates the growing importance of social media," says NPHIC Communications Director Brad Christensen. "People are realizing the value of its immediacy. With the rise of smartphones, social networking is a finger tap away" (Townsend, 2015).

Organizational use of social media is expanding in both the private and public sectors. Some evidence suggests that social media is also being adopted in public health and health education settings. Government agencies are increasingly interested in using social media to distribute information at the national (Thackeray et al., 2012), state and local levels. U.S. federal agencies, for example, routinely use a variety of social media sites including Twitter, Facebook, YouTube, Flickr, and Instagram to enhance communication (Shpayher, 2014). The U.S. government uses several social media services (Bhattacharya et al., 2014; Herman,, 2014; Hoover 2012; Jaeger et al., 2012, pp. 13–14).

Similarly, a literature survey in Canada shows that health organizations use social media and have moved to more interactive methods. It is no surprise that a variety of Canadian healthcare organizations, including the Public Health Agency of Canada, and many regional health units, such as Toronto Public Health and Peel Public Health are adopting social media in their practices in a variety of ways (Newbold and Campos, 2011). Organizations establish pages for community outreach, patient education, marketing and crisis communications, thereby taking advantage of the rapid speed and engaging nature of these sites (Bennett, 2009; Newbold and Campos, 2011).

### *Increased use of surveillance tools in programs in order to locate discourse in the social media*

To help assess the public's fears concerns, scholars have suggested using web-based methodologies as an insight into public response to infectious disease outbreaks (Signorini et al., 2011; Tausczik et al., 2012). Organizations can use social media for syndrome surveillance by monitoring the frequency of searches related to a particular illness; enlisting the public to report infections or symptoms; and mapping outbreaks with new tools and data mined from existing social networking sites.

These types of methodologies are used with increasing frequency in medical contexts with informal surveillance systems, such as Google Flu Trends (Brownstein et al., 2009; Dukic et al., 2009; Dukic et al., 2012) or FluBreaks (Pervaiz et al., 2012).

According to Brownstein (2011), one of the developers of HealthMap:

> We are now in an era where epidemic intelligence flows not only through government hierarchies but also through informal channels … Collecting these sources provide a view of global health that is fundamentally different from that yielded by diseases reporting in traditional public health infrastructures.

Specifically, online data mining analyzes the public via social discourse trends, noting correlations between the search words people use online and current events. This approach, known as "Internet-based bio-surveillance," "digital disease detection," or "event-based surveillance," has been described and analyzed in the literature (Brownstein et al., 2009; Hartley et al., 2010; Hartley et al., 2013). In the context of outbreak communication, this simple discourse surveillance tool can be used to identify people's fears and concerns as the outbreak unfolds, at both local and international levels, even focusing on specific areas or specific group profiles. Data mining is crucial for locating trends in public health concerns regarding the outbreak and treatments recommended, such as vaccines and medications. It is likewise crucial for developing an appropriate response for facilitating communication with the public. Nevertheless, on the level of communication systems, it has not yet been widely implemented. Evidence for its usefulness is provided by several recent studies. For example, Tausczik et al. (2012) investigated the effectiveness of new web-based methodologies in assessing anxiety and information-seeking in response to the 2009 H1N1 outbreak by examining language use in weblogs, newspaper articles, and web-based information seeking. They concluded that these methodologies may be a useful early marker of public anxiety, and provide a new insight into public response to infectious disease outbreaks (Tausczik et al., 2012). Similarly, Signorini et al. (2011) found that estimates of influenza-like illness derived from tweets accurately track reported disease levels, and concluded that Twitter could be used as a measure of public concern about health-related events. These findings demonstrate that monitoring web-related activity provides a dynamic picture of the way the public responds to an outbreak and that fluctuations in public anxiety about the outbreak can be detected in online writing and search trends.

## The old spirit of the organizations still haunts the public sphere on the social media

Despite this impressive transformation, the organizations' use of social media is still in its infancy. While the literature indicates that health authorities, at the international, national and local levels, actively use social media such as Twitter and Facebook, it also shows that this use is still very limited, as these tools serve primarily for mass information dissemination (similar to the traditional mass media), instead of two-way dialog mechanisms (Neiger et al., 2013b; Thackeray et al., 2012; Thackeray et al., 2013). As Danforth, Doying, Merceron, and Kennedy (2010) note, "Although other research has shown that the public uses sites such as Twitter and Facebook to communicate in emergency situations, response agencies have been slow in tapping into this type of communication tool however." Thus, one-way communication continues to predominate in the discourse, despite the fact that since 2009, the textbooks of the organizations call for their increased involvement in the social media and for interactive discourse whose goal is to respond to the fears and concerns of the public (Jones, 2011). Some studies have found that while social media tools have been adopted by state and local health departments, their primary use involves one-way communication about personal health topics and about organization-related topics (Neiger, et al., 2013b; Thackeray et al., 2012; Thackeray et al., 2013).

In 2012, most of the local authorities who did use social media tended to use it for one-way communication, as a tool for disseminating information. On average, state public health departments (SHDs) made one post per day on social media sites, and this was primarily to distribute information; there was very little interaction with the public. SHDs have few followers or friends on their social media sites. The most common topics on posts and tweets related to maintaining health and avoiding disease. There is also evidence that local public health departments (LHDs) are starting to use Twitter to engage their audiences in conversations. As public health transitions to more dialogic conversation and engagement, Twitter's potential to help form partnerships with audiences and involve them as program participants may lead to action for improved health.

In 2015, social media were still used for one-way communication. Neiger et al. (2012) found that of all the authorities' tweets on Ebola, 78.6% were to distribute information; 22.5% were about preparedness; 20.8% were updates; and 10.3% were about events.

However, limiting social media use to one-way communication decreases its interactive capacity to engage audiences (Wong et al., 2015). In fact, engaging audiences in two-way, conversational communication is the central purpose of social media (Safko, 2012).

Heldman, Schindelar, and Weaver III (2013) examined different levels of engagement for public health communication and consider the potential risks, benefits, and challenges of embracing the social component in public health practice. Neiger et al. (2012) have noted that there is little evidence to indicate that social media are used adequately by public health organizations in ways that leverage the ability to have meaningful conversations with the public, a communication approach labeled social media engagement (Heldman et al., 2013).

Furthermore, most of the organizations use a single platform rather than a variety of platforms that could foment more dynamic discourse and engage a wider range of subpopulations (Bergeron et al., 2013; Neiger et al., 2013b). For example, in 2012, a study found that 605 of state public health departments (SHDs) reported using at least one application on the social media. However, most of those who reported using these applications posted only one status update (Thackeray et al., 2012). A 2013 study found that local health departments used social media platforms sparingly, although larger departments made greater use of social media than smaller ones (Harris et al., 2013). A more recent study, conducted in 2015, found that 287 out of 2,700 local authorities in the USA had Twitter accounts, meaning that 10% of U.S. local authorities use Twitter (Wong et al., 2015). However, the study found that of the 287, only 174 actually used their accounts at least once a day during the period in which the study was conducted.

Local health department Twitter accounts were followed by more organizations than individual users. Organizations tended to be health-focused, located in a state other than the local health department being followed, and from the *education, government, and non-profit sectors*. Individuals were likely to be local and not health-focused. Having a public information officer on staff, serving a larger population, and "tweeting" more frequently were associated with having a higher percentage of local followers (Harris et al., 2014).

While social media can be used to disseminate health information, it should also be used to create dialog and engage audiences in true multidirectional interactions. Engagement is a key element in mobilizing and building communities and the benefit of social media is not maximized unless it engages community members (Lovejoy and Saxton, 2012). In the context of health promotion and social media, engagement has been defined as connections between people that contribute to a common good (Neiger et al., 2012) and result in some type of action on behalf of the individual or organization (Neiger et al., 2013a). This implies a mutual awareness and interaction between public health organizations and their audiences that lead to mutually beneficial outcomes. It is possible that the difficulty in conducting two-way communication is caused by the fact that many of the followers in different platforms are organizations and health officials, rather than laypeople.

It has been shown that even when campaigns use new and social media, they focus on passing the message fast in a one-way communication flow, ignoring both the public's reactions and the discourse in the social media (Tamura and Fukuda, 2011; Taylor et al., 2012).

## Current challenges faced by authorities

In order to attempt to mitigate the gaps in the public sphere, some crucial questions regarding the organizations' use of the social media will be discussed.

### *How do we put the* social *in social media?*

One of the most important questions is put forward by Heldman et al. (2013) namely: how do we "put *social* in social media?" Existing and emerging social media channels and tools that allow users to connect with public health organizations and with one another should not be dismissed as passing fads or trends – social media have become ubiquitous (Heldman et al., 2013; Mays et al., 2011). Fox (2011) states:

> The social life of health information is robust. The online conversation about health is being driven forward by two forces: 1) the availability of

social tools and 2) the motivation, especially among people living with chronic conditions, to connect with each other.

Heldman et al. (2013) suggest that one of the strategies to encourage greater engagement is seeing the person behind the public health organization. This improves trust and credibility over time, by allowing users to talk to and with the person versus interacting with an impersonal organization. Their study also emphasizes the importance of social discourse in moving people to act. They claim that at its very core, engagement requires that users do something with the information – listen, share, create, act, respond, and ask. The ultimate goal is for audiences to take action to improve their health by practicing healthy behaviors. There is limited evidence that engaging in online communication positively impacts people's health (Chou et al., 2013; Neiger et al., 2013a); this does not mean that the potential for impact is not there, just that more inquiry is needed.

### How can we evaluate the effectiveness of the organizations' use of social media?

Another challenge is how to evaluate factors associated with the levels of health agency engagement on social media in a systematic way. Major challenges lie in adapting social media technologies, include logistical issues, such as perceived resistance of government organizations to change, as well as the procedures, policies, and manpower needed to launch and effectively maintain a social media presence (Newbold and Campos, 2011; Schein et al., 2010).

Most of the organizations invest monetary resources in creating platforms, obtaining surveillance systems, recruiting professionals and using them in the social media. Less, however, is invested in evaluating the efficacy of organizational involvement in the social media. Evaluating the organizations' use of the social media and their influence requires constructing a methodology that conforms to the language, platforms, and goals of the users.

Korda and Itani (2013) point out that evaluation and measurement of social media engagement need to be better studied to determine if meaningful engagement is actually occurring. Jürgens (2012) notes the many opportunities and methodological challenges of evaluating and studying social media, as do Moorhead et al. (2013). Their systematic review found that many social media studies have limited methods and are exploratory and descriptive in nature, reporting eight gaps in the literature that need to be addressed, including studies with larger sample sizes and more robust methodologies.

In order to formulate a methodology, we must recognize the goals of campaign organizers in the social media and the ways they use them. The lack of evidence guiding public health enterprises is also a major challenge, but in part results from the difficulty that exists in evaluating such complex campaigns that often use different and multiple aspects of social media for a number of objectives. Exacerbating this, the current delay in publishing evidence in credible health journals lags behind the constantly and rapidly changing social media landscape, making it uncertain that literature will even be relevant for public health units by the time it is published (Schein et al., 2010). Additionally, although literature supports the feasibility of public health campaigns that are delivered online and through social media, more data is needed to determine the real costs of implementing such a program (Bennett and Glasgow, 2009; Newbold and Campos, 2011).

In public health, the Centers for Disease Control and Prevention actively use social media (CDC, 2015). However, we lack data on social media adoption within broader public health settings, particularly state public health departments. For example, Bhattacharya et al. (2014) argue that few studies have focused on how health agencies use Twitter. The studies that do exist describe activity consistent with distributing information with little attention paid to engagement (Thackeray et al., 2012). One of the few studies on engagement via Twitter focuses on levels of engagement – low (have followers), medium (promote retweeting) and high (have offline interactions) (Neiger et al., 2013a). Another example is the lack of evaluation during the Ebola crisis.

Despite widespread utilization of social media during emergency events and the adoption of social media by LHDs, to our knowledge, there have been no studies examining social media use specifically by LHDs during disease outbreaks, including the 2014 West Africa Ebola epidemic (Wong et al., 2015).

Neiger et al. (2013b) emphasize that while initial studies have reported frequent distributions of social media applications used in public health settings, no studies reported to date have investigated how social media is used within public health to engage audiences and involve them in actions related to programs and services. Beyond formulating a methodology for evaluation, the literature raises the question of measuring the results. The federal government and others have proposed a series of social media metrics in an attempt to standardize social media measurement (Herman, 2013; The Conclave on Social Media Measurement Standards, 2012). Heldman et al. (2013) indicated that more studies are needed to refine and establish an effective set of measurement tools.

## What outcomes do organizations desire from social media use?

In order to carry out such an evaluation, organizations must first define desirable ends and outcomes. Should the results focus on media engagement per se? Can the outcomes be measured by the amount of times the public resorts to the sources? Are results measured by the compliance to the organizations' recommendations? Can the results be evaluated by how satisfied the users are with the organizations? Can the results be measured by diffusion of information through Internet users to additional users on other social media platforms? Can the results be measured by the degree to which an organization uses two-way communication?

## Two-way communication

Literature on risk communication has drawn attention to the use of Hizon's convergence communication approach between the communicator and the audience. However, the findings presented in the preceding chapters demonstrate that despite the increased presence of organizations on social media, communication is still largely one way. This raises the following questions: how can we facilitate two-way communication? Is the format of FAQs (Frequently Asked Questions) often found on organizational websites and Facebook pages too superficial to be conducive to real dialog? How can a representative of an organization hold conversations with several participants simultaneously, responding to responses that arise simultaneously on different platforms? Another question arises, relating to what Heldman et al. (2013) have discussed, namely, how to turn the dialog into a conversation between two people: "Seeing the person behind the public health organization improves trust and credibility over time."

## Transformation

The world of social media has contributed to a radical transformation in the relationship between government organizations and the public, as McNab (2009) attests:

> Until recently the predominant communication model was 'one' authority to 'many' – i.e. a health institution, the ministry of health or a journalist communicating to the public. Social media has changed the monologue to a dialogue, where anyone with ICT access can be a content creator and communicator.
>
> (McNab, 2009)

In recent years, there has been a shift towards social media being used not just as a platform to connect with friends and family but also as the first place where users are apprised of breaking news stories. Eysenbach claims that this is a process called "apomediation," which is, in his words:

> an information-seeking strategy where people rely less on traditional experts and authorities as gatekeepers, but instead receive guidance from ... agents which stand-by ... to guide a consumer to high quality information and services without being a prerequisite to obtain that information or service in the first place, and with limited individual power to alter or select the information being brokered.
>
> (Eysenbach, 2008, p. e.22)

In this case, the government institutions themselves are afforded the possibility of stepping in at this point, and into these more intimate, individualized settings.

The importance of engaging individuals in order to meet their needs rather than to manage or control them is discussed in the literature. Are the organizations prepared to share information with people rather than managing them? Yet, the question that arises goes beyond how to construct a two-way communication which affects the individual who receives answers to questions posed (about which more studies are needed). It concerns the organizations themselves: how would the discourse affect and transform the organizations and their policies?

## References

Asulin-Karutchi, B. (2015). Pregnancy birth babies mam. Available at: https://he-il.fa cebook.com/portal.mamy/posts/10153119497552399 (accessed October 11, 2015).

Bennett, E. (2009). HSNL update #6. February 23. Available at: Cache (accessed March 3, 2009).

Bennett, G. G., and Glasgow, R. E. (2009). The delivery of public health interventions via the Internet: Actualizing their potential. *Annual Review of Public Health*, 30, 273–292.

Bergeron, K., Davies, J., Hahn, S., Brankley, L., Dhaliwal, M., Williams, M. *et al.* (2013). *Case Study: The Adoption of Social Media at Three Ontario Public Health Units.* Guelph, ON: Wellington-Dufferin-Guelph Public Health.

Betsch, C., Renkewitz, F., Betsch, T., and Ulshofer, C. (2010). The influence of vaccine-critical websites on perceiving vaccination risks. *Journal of Health Psychology*, 15(3), 446–455.

Bhattacharya, S., Srinivasan, P., and Polgreen, P. (2014). Engagement with health agencies on Twitter. *PloS ONE*, 9(11), e112235.

Boyle, M. P., Schmierbach, M., Armstrong, C. L., McLeod, D. M., Shah, D. V., and Pan, Z. (2004). Information seeking and emotional reactions to the September 11 terrorist attacks. *Journalism and Mass Communication Quarterly*, 81(1), 155–167.

Brookes, T., and Khan, O. A. (2005). *Behind the Mask: How the World Survived SARS, the First Epidemic of the 21st Century.* Washington, DC: American Public Health Association.

Brownstein, J. (2011). Using social media for disease surveillance. Available at: http:// globalpublicsquare.blogs.cnn.com/2011/08/18/using-social-media-for-disease-sur veillance/ (accessed April 23, 2016).

Brownstein, J. S., Freifeld, C. C., and Madoff, L. C. (2009). Digital disease detection: harnessing the Web for public health surveillance. *The New England Journal of Medicine*, 360(21), 2153–2157.

Bults, M., Beaujean, D. J., Richardus, J. H., van Steenbergen, J. E., and Voeten, H. A. (2011). Pandemic influenza A (H1N1) vaccination in The Netherlands: Parental reasoning underlying child vaccination choices. *Vaccine*, 29(37), 6226–6235.

CDC. (2015). Social media at CDC. Available at: www.cdc.gov/socialmedia/ (accessed April 23, 2016).

Chew, C., and Eysenbach, G. (2010). Pandemics in the age of Twitter: Content analysis of Tweets during the 2009 H1N1 outbreak. *PLoS ONE* 5(11), e14118.

Chou, W. Y., Prestin, A., Lyons, C., and Wen, K. Y. (2013). Web 2.0 for health promotion: Reviewing the current evidence. *American Journal of Public Health*, 103(1), e9–e18.

CohnJr, S. K. (2010). *Cultures of Plague: Medical Thinking at the End of the Renaissance.* Oxford: Oxford University Press.

Cunnion, S. O. (2003). Pneumonia – China (Guangdong): RFI. Available at: www.promedmail.org/ (accessed October 7, 2015).

Danforth, E., Doying, A., Merceron, G., and Kennedy, L. (2010). Applying social science and public health methods to community-based pandemic planning. *Journal of Business Continuity and Emergency Planning,* 4(4), 375–390.

Davies, M. (2009). Swine flu as social media epidemic; CDC tweets calmly. Available at: www.nielsen.com/us/en/insights/news/2009/swine-flu-as-social-media-epidemic-cdc-tweets-calmly.html (accessed May 1, 2009).

Drexler, M. (2008). Safety net. *The Journal of Life Sciences,* April/May, 56–63.

Dukic, V., Lopes, H. F., and Polson, N. (2009). Tracking flu epidemics using Google flu trends and particle learning. Available at: http://papers.ssrn.com/sol3/papers.cfm?abstract_id=1513705 (accessed April 23, 2016).

Dukic, V., Lopes, H. F., and Polson, N. (2012). Tracking epidemics with Google Flu Trends data and a State-Space SEIR Model. *Journal of the American Statistical Association,* 107(500), 1410–1426.

Eysenbach, G. (2008). Medicine 2.0: Social networking, collaboration, participation, apomediation, and openness. *Journal of Medical Internet Research,* 10(3), e22.

Fox, S. (2011). The social life of health information, 2011. Available at: www.pewinternet.org/2011/05/12/the-social-life-of-health-information-2011/ (accessed April 23, 2016).

Fung, I. C., Fu, K. W., Ying, Y., Schaible, B., Hao, Y., Chan, C. H. et al. (2013). Chinese social media reaction to the MERS-CoV and avian influenza A (H7N9) outbreaks. *Infectious Diseases of Poverty,* 2(1), 1–12.

Fung, I. C., Tse, Z. T., Cheung, C. N., Miu, A. S., and Fu, K. W. (2014). Ebola and the social media. *The Lancet,* 384(9961), 2207.

Gu, H., Chen, B., Zhu, H., et al. (2014). Importance of Internet surveillance in public health emergency control and prevention: Evidence from a digital epidemiologic study during avian influenza A H7N9 outbreaks. *Journal of Medical Internet Research,* 16(1), e20.

Harris, J. K., Choucair, B., Maier, R. C., Jolani, N., and Bernhardt, J. M. (2014). Are public health organizations tweeting to the choir? Understanding local health department Twitter followership. *Journal of Medical Internet Research,* 16(2), e31.

Harris, J. K., Mueller, N. L., and Snider, D. (2013). Social media adoption in local health departments nationwide. *American Journal of Public Health,* 103(9), 1700–1707.

Härtl, G. (2013). Novel coronavirus: The challenge of communicating about a virus which one knows little about. *Eastern Mediterranean Health Journal,* 19(suppl.1), S26–S30.

Hartley, D. M., Nelson, N. P., Arthur, R. R., Barboza, P., Collier, N., Lightfoot, N. *et al.* (2013). An overview of Internet biosurveillance. *Clinical Microbiology and Infection,* 19(11), 1006–1013.

Hartley, D. M., Nelson, N. P., Walters, R., *et al.* (2010). Landscape of international event-based biosurveillance. *Emerging Health Threats Journal,* 3, e3.

Heldman, A. B., Schindelar, J., and WeaverIII, J. B. (2013). Social media engagement and public health communication: Implications for public health organizations being truly "social." *Public Health Reviews,* 35, 1–18.

Henrich, N., and Holmes, B. (2011). Communicating during a pandemic: Information the public wants about the disease and new vaccines and drugs. *Health Promotion Practice,* 12(4), 610–619.

Herman, J. (2013). Social media metrics for federal agencies. Available at: www.digita lgov.gov/2013/04/19/social-media-metrics-for-federal-agencies/ (accessed April 23, 2016).

Herman, J. (2014). U.S. gov releases new collaborative social media services. Available at: www.digitalgov.gov/2014/06/30/u-s-gov-releases-new-collaborative-social-media -services/ (accessed April 23, 2016).

Hoover, J. N. (2012). Top 14 government social media initiatives. Available at: www. informationweek.com/applications/top-14-government-social-media-initiatives/d/d-id/ 1102918? (accessed April 23, 2016).

Hughes, A. L., Palen, L., Sutton, J., Liu, S. B., and Vieweg, S. (2008). "Site-seeing" in disaster: An examination of on-line social convergence. Paper presented at the 5th International ISCRAM Conference, Washington, DC, May.

Jaeger, P. T., Bertot, J. C., and Shilton, K. (2012). Information policy and social media: Framing government-citizen Web 2.0 interactions. In C. G. Reddick and S. K. Aikins (Eds.), *Web 2.0 Technologies and Democratic Governance. Political, Policy and Management Implications*, (pp. 13–14). New York: Springer.

Jones, B. (2011). Mixed uptake of social media among public health specialists. *Bulletin of the World Health Organization*, 89(11), 784–785.

Jürgens, P. (2012). Communities of communication: Making sense of the "social" in social media. *Journal of Technology in Human Services*, 30(3–4), 186–203.

Kata, A. (2012). Anti-vaccine activists, Web 2.0, and the postmodern paradigm: An overview of tactics and tropes used online by the anti-vaccination movement. *Vaccine*, 30(25), 3778–3789.

Korda, H., and Itani, Z. (2013). Harnessing social media for health promotion and behavior change. *Health Promotion Practice*, 14(1), 15–23.

Lovejoy, K., and Saxton, G. D. (2012). Information, community, and action: How nonprofit organizations use social media. *Journal of Computer-Mediated Communication*, 17(3), 337–353.

Matthews, G. (February 19, 2015). 2015's biggest health story was broken by a doctor – not a reporter. Available at: http://mdigitallife.com/2015s-biggest-hea lth-story-was-broken-by-a-doctor-not-a-reporter/ (accessed April 22, 2016).

Mays, D., WeaverIII, J. B., and Bernhardt, J. M. (2011). New media in social marketing. In G. Hastings, K. Angus and C. Bryant (Eds.), *The Sage Handbook of Social Marketing* (pp. 178–190). London: Sage.

McNab, C. (2009). What social media offers to health professionals and citizens. *Bulletin of the World Health Organization*, 87(8), 566.

Merchant, R. M., Elmer, S., and Lurie, N. (2011). Integrating social media into emergency-preparedness efforts. *New England Journal of Medicine*, 365(4), 289–291.

Mileti, D. S., and Darlington, J. D. (1997). The role of searching in shaping reactions to earthquake risk information. *Social Problems*, 44(1), 89–103.

Moorhead, S. A., Hazlett, D. E., Harrison, L., Carroll, J. K., Irwin, A., and Hoving, C. (2013). A new dimension of health care: Systematic review of the uses, benefits, and limitations of social media for health communication. *Journal of Medical Internet Research*, 15(4), e85.

Neiger, B. L., Thackeray, R., Burton, S. H., Giraud-Carrier, C. G., and Fagen, M. C. (2013a). Evaluating social media's capacity to develop engaged audiences in health promotion settings: Use of Twitter metrics as a case study. *Health Promotion Practice*, 14(2), 157–162.

Neiger, B. L., Thackeray, R., Burton, S. H., Thackeray, C. R., and Reese, J. H. (2013b). Use of Twitter among local health departments: An analysis of information sharing, engagement, and action. *Journal of Medical Internet Research*, 15(8), e177.

Neiger, B. L., Thackeray, R., Van Wagenen, S. A., et al. (2012). Use of social media in health promotion: Purposes, key performance indicators, and evaluation metrics. *Health Promotion Practice*, 13(2), 159–164.

Newbold, K. B., and Campos, S. (2011). *Media and Social Media in Public Health Messages: A Systematic Review*. Hamilton, ON: McMaster Institute of Environment and Health.

Odlum, M., and Yoon, S. (2015). What can we learn about the Ebola outbreak from tweets? *American Journal of Infection Control*, 43(6), 563–571.

Pervaiz, F., Pervaiz, M., Abdur Rehman, N., and Saif, U. (2012). FluBreaks: Early epidemic detection from Google flu trends. *Journal of Medical Internet Research*, 14(5), e125.

Petrie, K. J., and Faasse, K. (2009). Monitoring public anxiety about flu. Available at: http://blogs.bmj.com/bmj/2009/06/11/keith-j-petrie-and-kate-faasse-monitoring-public-anxiety-about-flu/ (accessed April 22, 2016).

Reuters. (2016). Zika virus 'buzzing' on Facebook, Twitter . *The Times of India Tech*. February 4. Available at: http://timesofindia.indiatimes.com/tech/social/Zika-vir us-buzzing-on-Facebook-Twitter/articleshow/50852284.cms

Rodriguez-Morales, A. J., Castañeda-Hernández, D. M., and McGregor, A. (2015). What makes people talk about Ebola on social media? A retrospective analysis of Twitter use. *Travel Medicine and Infectious Disease*, 13(1), 100–101.

Rotem, L. G. (2015). SciVac a company who manufactures Hepatitis B vaccine announced on a recall. Online Discussion Forum/Blogs, available at: http://rotter. net/forum/scoops1/234424.shtml (accessed July 31, 2015).

Safko, L. (2012). *The Social Media Bible: Tactics, Tools and Strategies for Business Success* (3rd edition). Hoboken, NJ: John Wiley & Sons, Inc.

Samarajiva, R., and Gunawardene, N. (February 6, 2013). Crying wolf over disasters undermines future warnings. Available at: www.scidev.net/global/policy/opinion/ crying-wolf-over-disasters-undermines-future-warnings-.html (accessed April 22, 2016).

Schein, R., Wilson, K., and Keelan, J. (2010). *Literature Review on Effectiveness of the Use of Social Media: A Report for Peel Public Health*. Vancouver: National Collaborating Centre for Public Health.

Shpayher, J. (2014). Federal agencies. Available at: http://govsm.com/w/Federal_Agen cies (accessed April 23, 2016).

Signorini, A., Segre, A. M., and Polgreen, P. M. (2011). The use of Twitter to track levels of disease activity and public concern in the U.S. during the influenza A H1N1 pandemic. *PloS ONE*, 6(5), e19467.

State of Israel Ministry of Health. (2015a). Discontinuation of use and market recall of the Sci-B-Vac Hepatitis Vaccine. Available at: www.health.gov.il/English/News_a nd_Events/Spokespersons_Messages/Pages/29072015_3.aspx (accessed October 11, 2015).

State of Israel Ministry of Health. (2015b). Clarification regarding the Sci-B-Vac Hepatitis B Vaccine. Available at: www.health.gov.il/English/News_and_Events/Sp okespersons_Messages/Pages/02082015.aspx (accessed October 11, 2015).Stiegler, R., Tilley, S., and Parveen, T. (2011). Finding family and friends in the aftermath of a disaster using federated queries on social networks and websites Web systems evolution (WSE). Paper presented at the 13th IEEE International Symposium on Web Systems Evolution (WSE),Williamsburg, VI,September 2011.

Tamura, Y., and Fukuda, K. (2011). Earthquake in Japan. *The Lancet*, 377(9778), 1652.

Tausczik, Y., Faasse, K., Pennebaker, J. W., and Petrie, K. J. (2012). Public anxiety and information seeking following the H1N1 outbreak: Blogs, newspaper articles, and Wikipedia visits. *Health Communication*, 27(2), 179–185.

Taylor, M., Wells, G., Howell, G., and Raphael, B. (2012). The role of social media as psychological first aid as a support to community resilience building. *Australian Journal of Emergency Management*, 27(1), 20–26.

Thackeray, R., Neiger, B. L., Burton, S. H., and Thackeray, C. R. (2013). Analysis of the purpose of state health departments' tweets: Information sharing, engagement, and action. *Journal of Medical Internet Research*, 15(11), e255.

Thackeray, R., Neiger, B. L., Smith, A. K., and Van Wagenen, S. B. (2012). Adoption and use of social media among public health departments. *BMC Public Health*, 12, 242.

The Conclave on Social Media Measurement Standards. (2012). Available at: www.smmstandards.wix.com/smmstandards

Townsend, V. (2015). State health agencies increasingly adopt social media, but brace for pay-to-play future. Available at: www.astho.org/StatePublicHealth/State-Health-Agencies-Increasingly-Adopt-Social-Media-but-Brace-for-Pay-to-Play-Future/3-10-15/ (accessed April 23, 2016).

WHO. (2003a). Summary of probable SARS cases with onset of illness from 1 November 2002 to 31 July 2003. Available at: http://www.who.int/csr/sars/country/table2004_04_21/en/ (accessed October 7, 2015).

WHO. (2003b). SARS: Lessons from a new disease. In *The World Health Report 2003: Shaping the Future*. Geneva: World Health Organization.

WHO. (2014). WHO declares end of Ebola outbreak in Nigeria. Available at: www.who.int/mediacentre/news/statements/2014/nigeria-ends-ebola/en/ (accessed April 22, 2016).

Wong, R., Harris, J. K., Staub, M., and Bernhardt, J. M. (2015). Local health departments Tweeting about Ebola: Characteristics and messaging. *Journal of Public Health Management and Practice,* September 2.

Yu, V. L., and Madoff, L. C. (2004). ProMED-mail: An early warning system for emerging diseases. *Clinical Infectious Diseases*, 39(2), 227–232.

Zhang, E. X., Yang, Y., Di Shang, R., et al. (2015). Leveraging social networking sites for disease surveillance and public sensing: The case of the 2013 avian influenza A (H7N9) outbreak in China. *Western Pacific Surveillance and Response*, 6(2), 66 72.

Zhang, P., and Gao, D. (2014). Collective sensemaking in social media: A case study of the H7N9 flu pandemic in China. Paper presented at the iConference2014, Berlin.

# 3    Organizational Policy and Practice

Organizational policies created to manage infectious diseases manifest how health authorities throughout the world operate in three domains: law, education, and ethics. This chapter aims to examine not only how authorities operate in crisis situations, when they are called upon to intervene in order to save lives, but more particularly, how they function in each of these domains in the long term. The chapter will unveil how, while preventative hygiene education has been neglected for many years, health authorities focus their efforts primarily on the legal arena, in which regulatory policy is sometimes contrived as voluntary. Regarding the domain of ethics, growing concerns about conflicts of interest (COIs) that stem from the symbiotic relationships between health authorities and the pharmaceutical industry will be discussed. The chapter will also discuss the industry's potential influence on decisions made by health authorities.

## Part 1 Educating the public in preventative hygiene

Dr. Ignaz Philipp Semmelweis, a Hungarian gynecologist, is described today as the "savior of mothers" and the father of infection control. In the mid-19th century, he made one of the most important contributions to modern medicine when he enforced a mandatory handwashing policy in the obstetric clinic in a Vienna hospital, and managed to dramatically decrease post-delivery mortality. Every morning, when Dr. Semmelweis, who had been appointed an assistant in obstetrics, visited his patients in the maternity ward, he heard their heart-breaking pleas. The women in labor were begging to be released and give birth anywhere else, even in the streets, just not in the hospital (Ataman et al., 2013). The year was 1847. At that time, about five women in 1,000 died in deliveries performed at home. Oddly, the post-delivery mortality at the best hospitals in Europe and America was often 10–20 times higher (Ataman et al., 2013; Markel, 2015). Semmelweis observed that in his hospital there was a tremendous difference in the rates of post-delivery mortality between women delivered by midwives, and those delivered by physicians and medical students. While the average death rate in the first group was 2%, the rate among women delivered by physicians and medical students was considerably higher, averaging 13%–18% (Best and Neuhauser, 2004). The reason for the mysterious deadly infection that struck the women, called puerperal fever or "childbed fever," was unknown. One of the most popular theories suggested it was miasmas – a harmful component in the air (Best and Neuhauser, 2004). Other explanations included poor ventilation, overcrowding, and the onset of lactation. Nevertheless, the prevailing view was that the disease was unpreventable (Markel, 2015).

Semmelweis could not agree with this defeatist conclusion. After considering several hypotheses, he concluded that the higher death rates in women delivered by medical students and their professors were associated with the autopsies they performed with their hands bare, before examining the laboring women (Best and Neuhauser, 2004). He instituted handwashing, using a chloride of lime solution, and in a controlled study managed to drastically reduce mortality rate to 2% – the same level as the midwives. Nonetheless, his superiors did not accept this idea, and in 1850, Semmelweis left Vienna and returned to his native Budapest. He was appointed as head physician of the obstetric ward of Pest's small St. Rochus Hospital, where he practically eliminated puerperal fever (Ellis, 2008). He later published various studies, indicating handwashing reduced mortality to below 1% (Best and Neuhauser, 2004).

Yet, despite this success, the medical community continued to reject his ideas, which challenged the established scientific opinions of the time. Two decades after his death, when Louis Pasteur, Koch, and Lister confirmed the germ theory, his work finally earned widespread acceptance (Ataman et al., 2013; Best and Neuhauser, 2004).

Today, hand hygiene is considered the most effective intervention for reducing infectious diseases and preventing the spread of antimicrobial resistance (Stewardson et al., 2011, p. 855). Moreover, sentences such as this open most publications regarding hand hygiene in the medical literature (Stewardson et al., 2011). The growing understanding that antiviral drugs and vaccination may not be enough to prevent catastrophe in the event of an epidemic (Jefferson et al., 2010; Jefferson et al., 2011), has led health organizations to advocate hand hygiene to both healthcare professionals and the public (CDC, 2015; WHO, 2009). For instance, according to the CDC, handwashing is like a "do-it-yourself" vaccine (CDC, 2015). In 2008, the Global Public-Private Partnership for Handwashing designated October 15 as Global Handwashing Day (GHD) in a campaign to motivate and mobilize people around the world to improve their handwashing habits by washing their hands with soap at critical moments each day. Since then, each year, October 15 is dedicated to awareness of handwashing with soap as a key approach to disease prevention (PPPHW, 2015). Indeed, systematic reviews conducted in the recent decade repeatedly indicate that the highest quality randomized controlled trials suggest respiratory virus spread can be prevented by handwashing (Jefferson et al., 2007; Jefferson et al., 2008; Jefferson et al., 2009; Jefferson et al., 2010; Jefferson et al., 2011). Moreover, a mounting body of evidence indicates that handwashing education, i.e., educating the public about the importance of handwashing and how to wash hands *correctly* and *at the correct time*, can significantly improve compliance, including among children (Azor-Martinez et al., 2014; Lau et al., 2012). More importantly, it can reduce risk of infectious disease (Azor-Martinez et al., 2014; Bloomfield et al., 2007; Lau et al., 2012; Little et al., 2015). For example, Little et al. (2015) used an internet intervention designed to increase handwashing, and demonstrated the effectiveness of such interventions in reducing the transmission of respiratory infections. Their study indicated that the risk of coming down with a respiratory tract infections was about 20% lower in the group that used the web-based program compared to the control group. The need for primary care consultations and antibiotic prescriptions was reduced by 10–15% in this group. Despite this evidence, the recent decade has witnessed a growing debate regarding the efficacy of handwashing, and scholars have argued that there is little evidence from randomized trials, especially among adults in non-deprived settings (Little et al., 2015). Indeed, the systematic reviews conducted by Jefferson et al. (Jefferson et al., 2007; Jefferson et al., 2008; Jefferson et al., 2009; Jefferson et al., 2010; Jefferson et al., 2011) indicate that the quality of some of the randomized controlled trials (RCTs) was poor and the risk of bias in them was high, as was the case for most cluster RCTs. The observational studies were of mixed quality, and only case-control data were sufficiently homogeneous to allow meta-analysis. Examining some of the studies reveals severe limitations that detract from the ability to draw reliable conclusions. For instance, Cowling et al. (2009) found that hand hygiene seemed to reduce influenza transmission, but the differences between the intervention and control group were not significant. Yet, the intervention in this study – hand hygiene with or without facemasks – was carried out among contacts in households that already had confirmed influenza virus infection. The delay from index patient symptom onset to intervention may have mitigated the effectiveness of handwashing. Another problem found in other studies is that for some reason, handwashing was not examined as a separate factor, but rather, hand hygiene was coupled with hand hygiene in the intervention group (Aiello et al., 2012; bin-Reza et al., 2012).

What are the implications of the debate on policies regarding widespread education for handwashing? It seems that the mere existence of this debate, 165 years after Dr. Semmelweis provided compelling evidence for the effectiveness of handwashing in preventing life-threatening infections, speaks for itself. The very fact that 150 years after the scientific community finally recognized its importance, there is still little evidence from good randomized trials regarding the effectiveness of this simple and low-cost practice, speaks for itself. Despite the fact that systematic reviews consistently indicate its effectiveness, and despite new evidence that makes clear that educating the public about the importance of handwashing and how to wash hands correctly and at the correct time is the key to achieve efficacy, still, too little has been done to increase awareness and education. An awareness day to increase handwashing is important, but it is hardly enough. As Jefferson et al. (2009) have indicated, more resources should be invested in research and in education for handwashing.

## Part 2 Vaccine policies

Immunization is considered one of the most effective tools available to prevent infectious diseases and their ensuing complications (Ada and Isaacs, 2000; Andre et al., 2008; Isaacs, 2012; Omer et al., 2009;). Indeed, in cases of rampant deadly outbreaks, such as the current Ebola epidemic, an efficient vaccine can save the lives of millions. At the same time, there is growing criticism of the policies of health authorities in various countries that aim to increase vaccination rates and to monitor and control immunization.

Ever since the first vaccines were introduced, there have been concerns about the increased risk of infectious disease outbreaks due to anti-vaccination attitudes and parents' refusal to vaccinate their children (Flanagan-Klygis et al., 2005; Simpson et al., 1995; Smith et al., 2004). This has led authorities worldwide to develop policies and legislation to confront these phenomena. In the USA, the first law mandating smallpox vaccination was passed in 1809 in Massachusetts, shortly after this first vaccine was introduced in America (Colgrove and Bayer, 2005; Orenstein and Hinman, 1999). Subsequently, other states endorsed similar legislations (Jackson, 1969). In a 1905 landmark case, *Jacobson v. Massachusetts*, the U.S. Supreme Court granted states the constitutional right to pass and enforce compulsory vaccination laws. In this case, the plaintiff, Pastor Henning Jacobson appealed to the U.S. Supreme Court, claiming that the fine imposed on him as a penalty for not complying with the City of Cambridge's mandatory smallpox vaccination was unconstitutional. The Court rejected the argument, insisting that in the face of epidemic, vaccination was a measure to eradicate smallpox (United States Supreme Court, 1905). The decision articulated the view that the state's interest in protecting the common welfare sometimes overrides the freedom of the individual (Mariner et al., 2005; Omer et al., 2009; Richins, 2011). In England, the Vaccination Act of 1853 mandated smallpox vaccination for all infants in the first three months of life. Parents who avoided compliance faced fines or prison (Daintith, 2008; Wolfe and Sharp, 2002). The Act of 1867 extended the compulsory immunization requirement to age 14, with cumulative penalties for non-compliance. These laws, in both the USA and England, represented a political innovation that extended government powers into areas of traditional civil liberties in the name of public health (Porter and Porter, 1988).

### *Immunization policies: from paternalism to voluntary models*

Today, immunization policies range from the most stringent paternalism to more voluntary models. Paternalistic policies are expressed in mandatory immunization.

According to a survey conducted as part of the VENICE project (Vaccine European New Integrated Collaboration Effort) among the 27 EU countries plus Iceland and Norway, 14 of these countries have at least one mandatory vaccination included in their program (Haverkate et al., 2012). Some of the countries demonstrate the toughest paternalism, mandating the vast part of the vaccines in their immunization programs. For example, Bulgaria, Hungary, Latvia, Poland, Slovaki,a and Romania have nine mandatory vaccines. At the opposite end of the spectrum are countries such as the UK, in which voluntary immunization policy is practiced.

Halfway between mandatory and voluntary immunization policies are policy types, which can be considered as "half-measure" or "semi-mandatory," such as policies barring unvaccinated children from attending public schools and/or monetary sanction policies.

Barring unvaccinated children from attending public schools is a practice that has been enforced in the USA since the 1920s. In 1922, in the case of *Zucht v. King*, the U.S. Supreme Court determined that states had substantial power to protect children from infectious disease, including not allowing them to attend public school (Parkins, 2012). Since then, courts have maintained the constitutionality of "government mandates for vaccination as a prerequisite for public school attendance" (Silverman, 2003), and by the beginning of the 1980s, all 50 states had school immunization requirements (Omer et al., 2009). Today, these laws often apply not only to children attending public school but also to those attending private school and day care (CDC, 2016).

A similar policy exists today in New Zealand, where a voluntary policy was practiced until the 1990s. Since 1995, any child in New Zealand attending early childhood centers and schools has been required to produce an immunization certificate that indicates whether he/she has been vaccinated (Dew, 1999).

Monetary sanction policies make continued financial assistance to families contingent on adherence to vaccination programs. Such sanctions may range from decreasing the amount of assistance to loss of benefits (Task Force, 2015). Studies that examined the effectiveness of monetary sanction policies to increase vaccination rates in children yielded conflicting evidence, as some indicated an increase in childhood immunization rates (Kerpelman et al., 2000), while others found no improvement in the vaccination rate (Minkovitz et al., 1999). A systematic review conducted by the Community Preventive Services Task Force in the USA found insufficient evidence to determine the effectiveness of monetary sanction policies to increase vaccination rates (Task Force, 2015). Nonetheless, some countries have recently revised their policies to introduce legislation that backs vaccination by welfare sanctions. For instance, in September 2015, the Australian government introduced a "no job, no pay" law, to prevent parents who refuse to vaccinate their children from receiving some government benefits (AAP, 2015).

In order to reduce public backlash, semi-mandatory policies usually offer various exemptions. For instance, in the USA, all states provide medical exemptions, and some state laws also offer exemptions for religious and/or philosophical reasons (CDC, 2016). These exemptions allow parents wide opt-outs of the mandate without expressing an objection to the policy itself, thus minimizing criticism. At the same time, there are voices calling to abolish the window that allows exemptions. In Australia, a new policy has already removed philosophical exemptions as of January 2016 (AAP, 2015). In the USA, a new Bill – Bill 277 (SB277), which was passed in the California State Senate in June 2015 and signed by Governor Jerry Brown on June 30, 2015 (Haelle, 2015), eliminated all exemptions from vaccine requirements for school entry except those medically indicated (Legislative Counsel Bureau State of California, 2015). Another new Bill that was assigned to a Congressional committee on May 1, 2015, *H.R. 2232: Vaccinate All Children Act of 2015,* suggests prohibiting the government from awarding preventive health-related grants to state institutions unless that state required all public school students to be vaccinated (U.S. Congress, 2015).

### Mandating vaccination policies and "herd immunity"

The rational justification that mandates or "semi-mandates" vaccination policies is based on health authorities' concerns regarding vaccine refusal as a significant obstacle to disease eradication (Saint-Victor and Omer, 2013). However, studies increasingly reveal that direct opposition to vaccination is actually a marginal phenomenon (Jacobson, 2010), and that in recent years, absolute refusal and anti-vaccination attitudes are gradually being replaced by a trend often defined as "vaccination hesitancy" (Diekema, 2012; Jacobson, 2010; Smith and Marshall, 2010). This trend, in which the benefits and dangers of vaccines are evaluated rationally (Jacobson, 2010; Velan et al., 2012), is reflected in the growing number of parents who delay vaccination of their children or refuse selected vaccines. Although compliance with immunization programs is generally high even in countries where vaccination is voluntary (Haverkate et al., 2012), health authorities argue that the phenomenon of vaccine hesitancy has led to a significant decrease in vaccination, which in its turn leads to a resurgence of outbreaks of vaccine-preventable diseases (Gowda and Dempsey, 2013). Without widespread compliance, they maintain, vaccines have a limited impact on public health (Saint-Victor and Omer, 2013).

A key term in this context is "herd immunity." Herd immunity is based on the assumption that "any given individual's chances of getting an infectious disease fall when others in society are immune because of previous vaccinations" (Kenkel, 2000, pp. 1677, 1694). According to Parkins (2012), if enough people in a community are vaccinated, their collective immunity eliminates the chains of contagion so that vulnerable members are protected from disease by the rest of the community. When a critical proportion of the population becomes immune, this is called the herd immunity threshold (HIT) or herd immunity level (HIL), then the disease no longer persists in this population, ceasing to be endemic (Rodpothong and Auewarakul, 2012, pp. 58–59; Somerville et al., 2012).

*Voluntary immunization policies: a true dialog or a pretense for patronizing policy instrument?*

How should health authorities implement immunization programs in a manner that would help maintain high vaccination rates, on one hand, and, on the other, be ethically justifiable? Several scholars have discussed this question, and stressed the importance of basing principles and operation of immunization programs on sound ethical values (Bradley, 1999; Isaacs, 2012; Verweij and Dawson, 2004), as well as on a dialog built on mutual respect between different perspectives on immunization (Vernon, 2003). Feudtner and Marcuse (2001) argue that public dialog is necessary to sustain consensus on immunization practices. According to Bradley (1999), in countries where high levels of population immunity exist, compulsory vaccination cannot, with very few exceptions, be justified. Isaacs (2012) further argues that compulsory vaccination can be ethically justified only as a last resort in special circumstances, such as the emergence of a devastating, new, vaccine-preventable disease, if the disease is sufficiently severe and if the vaccine is safe and effective.

The importance of promoting dialog as a means of building the public's trust in the authorities and in the immunization programs is endorsed by health authorities themselves. For example, in a document on communicating immunization entitled "Communication on immunization – building trust" (ECDC, 2012, p. 5), the ECDC stresses, "Dialogue is a vital ingredient in building trust, sharing knowledge and ensuring mutual understanding." Similarly, in a report on vaccine hesitancy, the WHO Strategic Advisory Group of Experts (SAGE) states: "Communication is increasingly about dialogue back and forth in the context of social media" (SAGE, 2014, p. 48).

But is the communication and the discourse regarding vaccines and immunization programs a true dialog? It has been argued that even in countries with voluntary immunization policies, the discourse used by health authorities to encourage parents to vaccinate their children is in fact far from genuine dialog based on mutual respect. Rather, it is a patronizing policy instrument, designed to generate discursive legitimacy for mass vaccination (Connell and Hunt, 2010; Dew, 1999). Such a discourse ostensibly preserves individual freedom (i.e., parents) regarding vaccines, and frames it as an "informed choice," but in fact, the rhetoric of "informed choice" serves as a means of obscuring the real message: that it is actually our duty as "responsible" parents to make not just an informed choice, but rather, the "right informed choice" (Dew, 1999).

The authorities' coercive discourse is based on various strategies, to be discussed in detail in Chapter 4. One example is intimidation. An example of an intimidating message is the message delivered by the New Zealand Health Ministry during a measles outbreak in 1997. The message stated: "You have a choice. Talk to your doctor about free immunization and remove the risk of measles forever. Or pray your child doesn't join the dots," and its implication, according to Dew, was clear: "Have your child vaccinated or risk their death from a brain-pulsating condition of encephalitis" (Dew, 1999, p. 388).

Furthermore, the parental responsibility is framed not just as individual responsibility for their own children, but as a civic duty, in order to maintain herd immunity. The Polio Vaccination Campaign in Israel, during a polio outbreak in 2013, is a good example. The campaign had a double message. On one hand, the Ministry of Health prompted parents to act responsibly and "Definitely vaccinate their children," since "A wild polio virus has broken out in Israel, which can cause paralysis and even death. The risk of the disease is real and tangible and not likely to disappear if children are not vaccinated" (State of Israel Ministry of Health, 2013).

On the other hand, alongside this message of parental responsibility, the vaccine was framed as a "social vaccine," and Health Ministry representatives explained that even children who had received the IPV vaccine and were therefore already vaccinated against the disease (all infants in Israel receive the IPV under the vaccination program), should receive the OPV as well. It was explained that this was the only way to protect those with weak immune systems and to achieve herd immunity, thereby eliminating the virus. Thus, the implication of this message was that part of parents' responsibility towards society is to vaccinate their children (Gal, 2013).

Similarly, Dew describes how during the 1991 measles epidemic, concerns were expressed that those who lower the herd immunity foster the spread of epidemics and, as such, become threats to the community (Dew, 1999).

Both of these "responsibility" framings – parents' "private" responsibility to protect their children by vaccinating them, and their "social" responsibility to maintain herd immunity, are depicted as complementary, and thus, when opposition is voiced to a particular vaccine or to the vaccination program, they are framed as threatening "herd immunity."

According to Connell and Hunt (2010), this type of coercive discourse constitutes a moral regulation project, directed at regulating both the self and others. That is, the control of the state over the individual is embodied in the project of voluntary mass vaccination, and the "informed choice" discourse serves as a powerful means that lends this practice moral legitimacy – a choice to be a responsible parent and civilian. Thus, in classically panoptic imagery, the public aligns itself with the governmental immunization programs without any need to mandate them (Dew, 1999).

The development of mass vaccination programs can be located in Foucault's concept of bio-politics (Connell and Hunt, 2010; Dew, 1999). According to Foucault, bio-politics is defined as practices of governing designed to control and supervise biological processes, such as propagation, births and mortality, health, life expectancy, and longevity. "Their supervision having been effected through an entire series of interventions and *regulatory controls: a bio-politics of the population*" (Foucault, 1978, p. 139; emphasis in original). These biological processes become regulated through a series of interventions and regulatory controls.

The focus of these practices is on populations, rather than on individuals. This strengthens the state (Foucault, 1988, p. 153). It is important to note that instead of relying on legislation, bio-politics relies on indirect control through self-regulation – imposing conformity with official policies (Dew, 1999). People's lives are managed and knowledge is derived from them through a system of surveillance and normalization of bodies. Thus, vaccine-preventable diseases become a threat, and therefore intervention and regulation must be imposed upon the body to normalize all bodies and make them immune to the disease. Moreover, in a further transition, instead of the virus, individuals who might transmit it become the primary source of danger, and therefore the individual must be controlled (Dew, 1999).

Yet, coercive discourse is not the only means health authorities use to achieve control. As some cases illustrate, there are also more "practical" means to impose vaccination even in countries with voluntary policies. While coercive discourse maintains at least a semblance of informed choice, even the option of seemingly "informed choice" is denied to parents. For instance, in Israel, the State Comptroller's Report for 2014 found that although babies in Israel receive their first vaccine (Hepatitis B vaccine) while still in the hospital, shortly after birth, their mothers do not receive information regarding the vaccine, or any other vaccine (The State Comptroller and Ombudsman of Israel, 2014, p. 619). Another way of curtailing parents' ability to make an "informed choice" is illustrated in the proceedings of the meeting of the Advisory Committee on Infectious Diseases and Immunizations of August 11, 2011. According to the proceedings, the committee discussed the presentation of vaccine side effects in the Ministry of Health publications on immunization, and decided that these publications should not include the full information regarding the side effects presented in the vaccine bulletins, but rather, a limited version, in which the information on vaccines from different manufacturers is processed, aggregated, and consolidated (State of Israel Ministry of Health, Haifa District Health Office, 2011).

Another way to reinforce the pretense of free choice is by performing vaccinations in schools, since, as was found in the case of the HPV vaccine, parents who refuse must be proactive and declare in writing that they do not want their child vaccinated (Gesser-Edelsburg et al., 2015). Furthermore, sometimes, parents who refuse vaccination are asked to state the reason in the consent forms (Stretch et al., 2008), which requires them to be even more proactive.

The processed and aggregated information presented in the Health Ministry's publications for parents, as well as in those consent forms parents are asked to sign also demonstrate what Lupton refers to as a "slippage" between education and indoctrination (Lupton, 1995, p. 110). This aggregated information becomes "facts," and the "facts" are conveyed as "true."

All these practices – the coercive discourse, as well as additional means taken to empower the coercion, which eliminate even the appearance of "informed choice" – result in an immunization program that although is considered voluntary, it in fact, verges on mandatory.

## Part 3 Conflict of interests

"A profit-driven industry does not invest in products for markets that cannot pay," asserted the WHO Director General Margaret Chan in a speech at a conference in the West African country of Benin, in the midst of the Ebola crisis. Criticizing the pharmaceutical industry, Chan claimed that its drive for profit was one of the reasons the development of an Ebola vaccine had been delayed. "Two WHO arguments that have fallen on deaf ears for decades are now out there with consequences that all the world can see, every day, on prime-time TV news" (Gladstone, 2014). Although focusing the blame on the industry, the WHO itself was criticized for its "collusive relations" with it, which was one of the problems that led, it was claimed, to the organization's inability to fight Ebola (*Sentaku* Magazine, 2014).

Brice de le Vingne, Director of Operations for Doctors without Borders, said that the WHO's position could be compared to a frog in a pot of water on a stove.

> If you put a frog in cold water and start to heat it, she will not jump out of the pan, she will adapt to the temperature and she will not realize that she is boiling to death. WHO is the same.
>
> (Hussain, 2014)

The criticism of the WHO's stance during the current Ebola epidemic reflects the growing concern regarding conflicts of interest and "collusions" between health authorities and pharmaceutical companies, and regarding the potential influence of the pharmaceutical industry on the decisions made by health authorities (Cohen and Carter, 2010; Epstein, 2011; Godlee, 2010; Social Health and Family Affairs Committee, 2010). As Resnik (2004) points out, COIs can lead to biased research, injuries, and low trust. But it can also lead to unbalanced allocation of budgets to diseases (Nozaki, 2013; Stuckler et al., 2008), and to a flawed approval process of drugs and vaccines (Cohen and Carter, 2010; DeLong, 2012; Ferner, 2005). Perhaps the most prominent example of this concern is the 2009 H1N1 outbreak. In the aftermath of the H1N1 outbreak, there were significant concerns about competing interests among experts on influential advisory committees, including the WHO Emergency Committee (Cohen and Carter, 2010; Epstein, 2011; Social Health and Family Affairs Committee, 2010). Members of the WHO Emergency Committee have been linked to manufacturers of both neuraminidase inhibitors and influenza vaccines (Cohen and Carter, 2010; Epstein, 2011). "This was a pandemic that never really was," claimed Paul Flynn, a U.K. politician charged with investigating the handling of the H1N1 outbreak for the Council of Europe (Macrae, 2010). On June 4, 2010, the Council of Europe Parliamentary Assembly published a harsh report (Social Health and Family Affairs Committee, 2010), claiming that the decision-making surrounding the H1N1 crisis has been lacking in transparency, had caused unjustified fear and had prompted countries around the world to waste millions of dollars.

According to the report:

> The parliamentary assembly is alarmed about the way in which the H1N1 influenza pandemic has been handled, not only by the WHO, but also by the competent health authorities at the level of the European Union and at national level. It is particularly troubled by some of the consequences of decisions taken and advice given leading to distortion of priorities of public health services across Europe, waste of large sums of public money, and also unjustified scares and fears about health risks faced by the European public at large.

Another report, a joint investigation by the *British Medical Journal* and the Bureau of Investigative Journalism (Cohen and Carter, 2010), uncovered evidence that raised troubling questions about how the WHO managed competing interests among the scientists who advised its pandemic planning, and about the transparency of the science underlying its advice to governments. According to the report, the 2004 guidelines the WHO developed were based in part on the advice of experts who received consulting fees from the two leading manufacturers of antiviral drugs used against the virus: Roche and GlaxoSmithKline. Yet these COIs have never been publicly disclosed by WHO. "We are left wondering whether major public health organizations are able to effectively manage the conflicts of interest that are inherent in medical science," wrote Cohen and Carter (2010, p. 1274). Their report detailed WHO's pandemic influenza preparation starting in 1999, when a preparedness plan was drafted by six researchers in collaboration with the European Scientific Working Group on Influenza (ESWI). According to the report, what that document did not disclose, was the fact that ESWI is funded entirely by Roche. Roche makes the influenza antiviral Tamiflu (oseltamivir). The USA alone had stockpiled nearly US$1.5 billion dollars worth of it prior to the 2009 H1N1 outbreak (Doshi et al., 2012).

Furthermore, in the events leading up to the 2009 pandemic, WHO did not reveal the identity of the 16 members of Emergency Committee who were to advise the WHO on its policy regarding the beginning and end of the 2009 pandemic (Social Health and Family Affairs Committee 2010). The members of this committee were not disclosed to the public (Cohen and Carter, 2010).

### Financial reliance on the pharmaceutical industry

A major issue at the center of the concerns around COIs is the authorities' heavy financial reliance on the pharmaceutical industry. According to Shah (2011), a group composed of business corporations, including Coca-Cola Co. and Pfizer Inc., is the world's top source of financing and leadership in the fight against deadly disease. As the WHO, starved of public financing, is forced to rely upon voluntary contributions, these corporations' donations constitute today nearly 80% of the agency's budget. Thus, they exert influence on the WHO's policies and decision-making, and shape the global health agenda. The result is reflected in the agency's allocation of budgets to diseases. While its regular budget is allocated to diseases that account for highest mortality around the world, most of the extra budgetary funds, which constitute the bulk of the WHO's overall expenditures, is spent on illnesses that account for a tiny fraction of global mortality (Shah, 2011). Diseases like malaria and tuberculosis, which together cause 2 million deaths a year, have received less attention from the WHO than high cholesterol (Surowiecki, 2014). According to Chirac and Torreele (2006), only 18 of the 1,556 new drugs that were developed between 1975 and 2004 were for tropical diseases that the pharmaceutical industry has neglected. This group of parasitic and bacterial diseases, such as Chagas disease and dengue, affects more than one billion people globally and kills an estimated 534,000 people worldwide every year (CDC, 2014).

Stuckler et al. (2008) reported that WHO budget allocations were heavily skewed towards control of infectious diseases. They concluded that WHO funding did not match the disease burden, particularly in the Western Pacific region, which has low rates of infectious diseases and a high burden of non-communicable diseases compared to Africa. A reassessment of WHO's budgetary allocation carried out five years later yielded similar results. In 2008–13, WHO's budgetary allocations were still heavily skewed towards control of infectious diseases both in Africa, and in the Western Pacific region (Nozaki, 2013).

COIs and industry funding could also result in industry influence on the approval process of drugs and vaccines (Cohen and Carter, 2010; DeLong, 2012; Ferner, 2005). Doshi (2013) argues that the studies underlying the U.S. policy promoting influenza vaccines, which he claims is one of the most visible and aggressive public health policies today, are often of low quality, and do not substantiate officials' claims. According to (DeLong, 2012), this policy is largely the result of the FDA's heavy reliance on the drug companies. The fees that the drug companies pay to the U.S. FDA to have their drugs evaluated (in accordance with the Prescription Drug User Fee Act, adopted in 1992), she argues, can influence the approval decisions. Although the Act refers only to prescription drugs and not vaccines, since many vaccine manufacturers also produce prescription drugs, the user fees paid by them provide incentives for the FDA to be friendlier towards them (DeLong, 2012). Similarly, in the UK, a report released by the House of Commons Health Committee on "the influence of the pharmaceutical industry," described the substantial impact of this industry on health authorities (Ferner, 2005). According to the report, the annual income of the Medicines and Healthcare Products Regulatory Agency (MHRA), which is the executive arm of the drugs Licensing Authority in the UK, stands at £65m, derived entirely from licensing fees.

The committee thought that the need to attract pharmaceutical business could conflict with the MHRA's duty to protect the public, and undermine the thoroughness with which the MHRA reviews data submitted for licensing, as well as its ability, after licensing, to detect adverse drug reactions and act on them. Cohen and Carter's (2010) report on the pandemic planning refers to the chain of approval of influenza drugs in the FDA and the EMEA. In the USA, the FDA Advisory Committee initially rejected Zanamivir, another influenza antiviral drug, because it lacked efficacy. But the FDA leadership overruled the committee and criticized its reviewer, biostatistician Michael Elashoff. The review of Oseltamivir, which was also undergoing the approval process at that time, was taken away from him, and reassigned to someone else (Cohen and Carter, 2010). In the EU, experts who provided opinions during the EMEA licensing process for Oseltamivir in 1999 had financial connections with Roche, the drug-maker (Cohen and Carter, 2010).

## *The revolving door*

Another major problem related to the COIs is the "revolving door" – the free movement of key employees between regulators and drug companies (Goldacre, 2013). Officials at government regulators may see working for the government as a stepping stone to a lucrative position at a drug company. For example, in January 2010, a year after leaving as Director of CDC – an agency charged with overseeing vaccines and drug companies, Dr. Julie Gerberding took up a position as president of Merck Vaccines. During her tenure as CDC Director from 2002 to 2008, Dr. Gerberding supported studies that concluded that no link between vaccines and neurological disorders could be found (DeLong, 2012). In January 2011, Elias Zerhouni, former Director of the NIH – one of the world's foremost medical research centers, and an agency of the U.S. Department of Health and Human Services – became the President of Sanofi-Aventis research and development, covering medicines and vaccines (Sanofi, 2010). This frequent exchange of personnel can create a further problem – what if those public officials, while working in a government agency, are more concerned with their future at a pharmaceutical company? It is possible that they might be reluctant to make decisions that would alienate a potential future employer (Goldacre, 2013). And while studies of these officials' conduct while still working for the government agency may be good analyses, the COI regarding research emphasis or conclusions is unavoidable when they move to the industry that they previously regulated (DeLong, 2012).

Similar to regulator employees, it was argued that scientific and medical experts advising the agencies and sitting on advisory boards often operate with a conflict of interest. For instance, Lurie, Almeida, Stine, Stine, and Wolfe (2006) found that conflicts of interest are common within FDA drug panels: in 2001–2004, a financial conflict of interest with the affected company was had by one or more panel members in 73% of the 221 drug reviews conducted by the FDA's 16 advisory committees. In a survey conducted among 997 scientists working at the FDA, 61% said they knew of cases where "Department of Health and Human Services or FDA political appointees have inappropriately injected themselves into FDA determinations or actions." Some 18.4%

said that they themselves "have been asked, for nonscientific reasons, to inappropriately exclude or alter technical information or their conclusions in an FDA scientific document" (Fromer, 2006).

In 2011, the Australian media revealed that Professor Anne Kelso, one of the WHO immunization advisers and the Director of the WHO Collaborating Centre for Reference and Research on Influenza, owns shares in CSL, Australia's sole manufacturer of flu vaccines (Bita, 2011). Nevertheless, according to a WHO report, "Based on the WHO assessment of the interest declared by Professor Kelso, it was concluded that Professor Kelso should continue to serve as an Adviser." According to the report, the decision was based on the fact that Kelso had disclosed her COI at the beginning of the consultation, and considering her agreement "to refrain from acquiring additional shares in companies involved in influenza vaccine manufacture" (WHO, 2015, p. 6).

Moreover, sometimes, COIs are not even disclosed. For example, in 2009, a U.S. Health and Human Services Inspector General's report found that "for almost all special Government employees, the CDC did not ensure that financial disclosure forms were complete in 2007." According to the report, the CDC certified financial disclosure forms with at least one omission in 2007 for 97% of committee members – and most of the forms had more than one type of omission. Furthermore, the report stated that 64% of the committee members had potential conflicts of interest in 2007 that CDC did not identify or resolve before certifying their forms (Levinson, 2009).

Similarly, in Israel, the State Comptroller's Report for 2014 found that the members of the Advisory Committee on Infectious Diseases and Immunizations do not always declare their conflicts of interest at the beginning of each meeting, although according to the terms of appointment, members of the committee and advisors are obliged to do so. The report also indicated that "the head of the committee asks its members to declare their COIs only when he has knowledge about a relationship between the members and a vaccine manufacturer, whose vaccine is to be discussed at that meeting" (The State Comptroller and Ombudsman of Israel, 2014, p. 623).

### Possible solutions

Goldacre (2013) uses the term "regulatory capture" to describe the process whereby health regulators end up promoting the interests of the industry they were supposed be monitoring, at the expense of the public interest. Ferner (2005) calls the health authorities "David," and argues that they stand very little chance of triumphing over the pharmaceutical "Goliath," as they have no resources to ensure their independence. But is that regulatory failure indeed doomed? How, if at all, can conflicts of interest be prevented? There are no easy solutions.

DeLong (2012) suggests closing the revolving door between regulators and drug manufacturers, so that officials could not use public service as a stepping stone to lucrative positions in private industries. Furthermore, she demands that any person in a vaccine policy-making position or any member of a vaccine advisory committee have no past funding or salary from a vaccine manufacturer, nor should they own stock in a vaccine company. But finding qualified vaccine experts who have no past ties to pharmaceutical companies can be very difficult (Drazen and Curfman, 2002). In order to succeed in the implementation of such policy, or achieve at least a partial success, the implementation process must be long term and each step must be considered carefully.

# References

AAP. (2015). Vaccination to be backed by welfare sanctions. *The Australian*. April 12. Available at: www.theaustralian.com.au/national-affairs/health/vaccination-to-be-ba cked-by-welfare-sanctions/news-story/6337528471b2b26bd2a5511602bd6903

Ada, G. L., and Isaacs, D. (2000). *Vaccination: The Facts, the Fears, the Future*. Sydney: Allen and Unwin.

Aiello, A. E., Perez, V., Coulborn, R. M., et al. (2012). Facemasks, hand hygiene, and influenza among young adults: A randomized intervention trial. *PLoS ONE*, 7(1), e29744.

Andre, F., Booy, R., Bock, H., et al. (2008). Vaccination greatly reduces disease, disability, death and inequity worldwide. *Bulletin of the World Health Organization*, 86 (2), 140–146.

Ataman, A. D., Vatanoğlu-Lutz, E. E., and Yıldırım, G. (2013). Medicine in stamps: Ignaz Semmelweis and puerperal fever. *Journal of the Turkish German Gynecological Association*, 14(1), 35–39.

Azor-Martinez, E., Cobos-Carrascosa, E., Gimcncz-Sanchez, F., et al. (2014). Effectiveness of a multifactorial handwashing program to reduce school absenteeism due to acute gastroenteritis. *The Pediatric Infectious Disease Journal*, 33(2), e34–e39.

Best, M., and Neuhauser, D. (2004). Ignaz Semmelweis and the birth of infection control. *Quality and Safety in Health Care*, 13(3), 233–234.

bin-Reza, F., Lopez Chavarrias, V., Nicoll, A., and Chamberland, M. E. (2012). The use of masks and respirators to prevent transmission of influenza: A systematic review of the scientific evidence. *Influenza and Other Respiratory Viruses*, 6(4), 257–267.

Bita, N. (2011). Flu adviser defends CSL shares. *The Australian*. September 8. Available at: www.theaustralian.com.au/national-affairs/flu-adviser-defends-csl-shares/story-fn59 niix-1226131711216

Bloomfield, S. F., Aiello, A. E., Cookson, B., O'Boyle, C., and Larson, E. L. (2007). The effectiveness of hand hygiene procedures in reducing the risks of infections in home and community settings including handwashing and alcohol-based hand sanitizers. *American Journal of Infection Control*, 35(10), Supplement 1, S27–S64.

Bradley, P. (1999). Should childhood immunisation be compulsory? *Journal of Medical Ethics*, 25(4), 330–334.

CDC. (2014). Neglected tropical diseases. Available at: www.cdc.gov/globalhealth/ntd/ (accessed April 27, 2016).

CDC. (2016). State vaccination requirements. Available at: www.cdc.gov/vaccines/im z-managers/laws/state-reqs.html (accessed January 29, 2016).

CDC. (2015). Handwashing: Clean hands save lives. Available at: www.cdc.gov/ha ndwashing/ (accessed April 24, 2015).

Chirac, P., and Torreele, E. (2006). Global framework on essential health R&D. *The Lancet*, 367(9522), 1560–1561.

Cohen, D., and Carter, P. (2010). WHO and the pandemic flu "conspiracies." *BMJ*, 340(7759), 1274–1279.

Colgrove, J., and Bayer, R. (2005). Could it happen here? Vaccine risk controversies and the specter of derailment. *Health Affairs*, 24(3), 729–739.

Connell, E., and Hunt, A. (2010). The HPV vaccination campaign: A project of moral regulation in an era of biopolitics. *Canadian Journal of Sociology*, 35(1), 63–82.

Cowling, B. J., Chan, K. H., Fang, V. J., Cheng, C. K. Y., Fung, R. O. P., Wai, W., et al. (2009). Facemasks and hand hygiene to prevent influenza transmission in households: A cluster randomized trial. *Annals of Internal Medicine*, 151(7), 437–446.

Daintith, J. (2008). *Biographical Encyclopedia of Scientists*. Boca Raton, FL: CRC Press.

DeLong, G. (2012). Conflicts of interest in vaccine safety research. *Accountability in Research: Policies and Quality Assurance*, 19(2), 65–88.

Dew, K. (1999). Epidemics, panic and power: Representations of measles and measles vaccines. *Health*, 3(4), 379–398.

Diekema, D. S. (2012). Issues leading to vaccine hesitancy. Paper presented at the Presentation to Meeting 2 of the Institute of Medicine Committee on the Assessment of Studies of Health Outcomes Related to the Recommended Childhood Immunization Schedule. Atlanta, GA.

Doshi, P. (2013). Influenza: Marketing vaccine by marketing disease. *BMJ*, 346, f3037.

Doshi, P., Jefferson, T., and Del Mar, C. (2012). The imperative to share clinical study reports: Recommendations from the Tamiflu experience. *PLoS Medicine*, 9(4), e1001201.

Drazen, J. M., and Curfman, G. D. (2002). Financial associations of authors. *New England Journal of Medicine*, 346(24), 1901–1902.

ECDC. (2012). *Communication on Immunisation: Building Trust*. Stockholm: European Centre for Disease Prevention and Control.

Ellis, H. (2008). Ignaz Semmelweis: Tragic pioneer in the prevention of puerperal sepsis. *British Journal of Hospital Medicine*, 69(6), 358.

Epstein, H. (2011). Flu warning: Beware the drug companies! Available at: www.nybooks.com/articles/2011/05/12/flu-warning-beware-drug-companies/ (accessed April 26, 2016).

Ferner, R. E. (2005). The influence of big pharma. *BMJ*, 330(7496), 855–856.

Feudtner, C., and Marcuse, E. K. (2001). Ethics and immunization policy: Promoting dialogue to sustain consensus. *Pediatrics*, 107(5), 1158–1164.

Flanagan-Klygis, E. A., Sharp, L., and Frader, J. E. (2005). Dismissing the family who refuses vaccines: A study of pediatrician attitudes. *Archives of Pediatrics and Adolescent Medicine*, 159(10), 929–934.

Foucault, M. (1978). *The History of Sexuality*. vol. I: *An Introduction* (trans. R. Hurley). New York: Pantheon Books.

Foucault, M. (1988). The political technology of individuals. In L. H. Martin, H. Gutman and P. H. Hutton (Eds.), *Technologies of the Self: A Seminar with Michel Foucault*. Amherst, MA: University of Massachusetts Press.

Fromer, M. J. (2006). Survey of FDA scientists shows they feel pressure to exclude or alter findings fear retaliation for voicing safety concerns. *Oncology Times*, 28(16), 12–13, 16.

Gal, I. (2013). Social vaccine: the child is protected from polio – Why vaccinate? *YNET*. Available at: www.ynet.co.il/articles/0,7340,L-4416155,00.html

Gesser-Edelsburg, A., Walter, N., Shir-Raz, Y., and Green, M. S. (2015). Voluntary or mandatory? The valence framing effect of attitudes regarding HPV vaccination. *Journal of Health Communication*, 20(11), 1287–1293.

Gladstone, R. (2014). W.H.O. assails delay in Ebola vaccine . *The New York Times*, November 3. Available at: www.nytimes.com/2014/11/04/world/africa/ebola-cur e-delayed-by-drug-industrys-drive-for-profit-who-leader-says.html?_r=3

Godlee, F. (2010). Conflicts of interest and pandemic flu. *BMJ*, 340, c2947.

Goldacre, B. (2013). *Bad Pharma: How Drug Companies Mislead Doctors and Harm Patients*. New York: Faber and Faber.

Gowda, C., and Dempsey, A. F. (2013). The rise (and fall?) of parental vaccine hesitancy. *Human Vaccines and Immunotherapeutics*, 9(8), 1755–1762.

Haelle, T. (2015). California Vaccination Bill SB 277 signed by governor, becomes law. *Forbes*, June 30,

Haverkate, M., D'Ancona, F., Giambi, C., *et al.* (2012). Mandatory and recommended vaccination in the EU, Iceland and Norway: Results of the VENICE 2010 survey on the ways of implementing national vaccination programmes. Available at: www.eurosurveillance.org/images/dynamic/EE/V17N22/art20183.pdf

Hussain, M. (2014). Ebola response of MSF and 'boiling frog' WHO under scrutiny. *Reuters*. August 21.

Isaacs, D. (2012). An ethical framework for public health immunisation programs. *New South Wales Public Health Bulletin*, 23(6), 111–115.

Jackson, C. L. (1969). State laws on compulsory immunization in the United States: A review. *Public Health Reports*, 84(9), 787–795.

Jacobson, R. M. (2010). Vaccination refusal and parental education: Lessons learnt and future challenges. *Pediatric Health*, 4(3), 239–242.

Jefferson, T., Del Mar, C., Dooley, L., *et al.* (2009). Physical interventions to interrupt or reduce the spread of respiratory viruses: Systematic review. *BMJ*, 339, b3675.

Jefferson, T., Del Mar, C., Dooley, L., et al. (2010). Physical interventions to interrupt or reduce the spread of respiratory viruses. *Cochrane Database of Systematic Reviews*, 20(1).

Jefferson, T., Del Mar, C. B., Dooley, L., et al. (2011). Physical interventions to interrupt or reduce the spread of respiratory viruses. *Cochrane Database of Systematic Reviews*, 6(7).

Jefferson, T., Foxlee, R., Del Mar, C., et al. (2007). Interventions for the interruption or reduction of the spread of respiratory viruses. *Cochrane Database of Systematic Reviews*, 4.

Jefferson, T., Foxlee, R., Mar, C. D., et al. (2008). Physical interventions to interrupt or reduce the spread of respiratory viruses: Systematic review. *BMJ*, 336(7635), 77–80.

Kenkel, D. S. (2000). Prevention. In A. J. Culyer and J. P. Newhouse (Eds.), *Handbook of Health Economics* (Vol. 1, pp. 1675–1720). Oxford: Elsevier.

Kerpelman, L. C., Connell, D. B., and Gunn, W. J. (2000). Effect of a monetary sanction on immunization rates of recipients of aid to families with dependent children. *JAMA*, 284(1), 53–59.

Lau, C. H., Springston, E. E., Sohn, M. W., *et al.* (2012). Hand hygiene instruction decreases illness-related absenteeism in elementary schools: A prospective cohort study. *BMC Pediatrics*, 12(52), 1–7.

Legislative Counsel Bureau State of California. (2015). Senate Bill No. 277, Public health: vaccinations. June 30. Available at: http://leginfo.legislature.ca.gov/faces/ billNavClient.xhtml?bill_id=201520160SB277.

Levinson, D. R. (2009). *CDC's Ethics Program for Special Government Employees on Federal Advisory Committees*. Washington, DC: Department of Health and Human Services. Office of Inspector General.

Little, P., Stuart, B., Hobbs, F. D. R., Moore, M., Barnett, J., Popoola, D., et al. (2015). An internet-delivered handwashing intervention to modify influenza-like illness and respiratory infection transmission (PRIMIT): A primary care randomised trial. *The Lancet*, 386(10004), 1631–1639.

Lupton, D. (1995). *The Imperative of Health: Public Health and the Regulated Body*. London: Sage.

Lurie, P., Almeida, C. M., Stine, N., Stine, A. R., and Wolfe, S. M. (2006). Financial conflict of interest disclosure and voting patterns at Food and Drug Administration Drug Advisory Committee meetings. *JAMA*, 295(16), 1921–1928.

Macrae, F. (2010). The pandemic that never was: Drug firms 'encouraged world health body to exaggerate swine flu threat'. *Daily Mail*, June 4. Available at: www.dailymail.co.uk/news/article-1284133/The-pandemic-Drug-firms-encouraged-world-health-body-exaggerate-swine-flu-threat.html

Mariner, W. K., Annas, G. J., and Glantz, L. H. (2005). Jacobson v Massachusetts: It's not your great-great-grandfather's public health law. *American Journal of Public Health*, 95(4), 581–590.

Markel, H. (2015). In 1850, Ignaz Semmelweis saved lives with three words: wash your hands. Available at: www.pbs.org/newshour/updates/ignaz-semmelweis-doctor-prescribed-hand-washing/ (accessed April 24, 2016).

Minkovitz, C., Holt, E., Hughart, N., *et al.* (1999). The effect of parental monetary sanctions on the vaccination status of young children: An evaluation of welfare reform in Maryland. *Archives of Pediatrics and Adolescent Medicine*, 153(12), 1242–1247.

Nozaki, I. (2013). WHO's budgetary allocation and disease burden. *The Lancet*, 382 (9896), 937–938.

Omer, S. B., Salmon, D. A., et al. (2009). Vaccine refusal, mandatory immunization, and the risks of vaccine-preventable diseases. *New England Journal of Medicine*, 360(19), 1981–1988.

Orenstein, W. A., and Hinman, A. R. (1999). The immunization system in the United States – The role of school immunization laws. *Vaccine*, 17(Supplement 3), S19–S24.

Parkins, C. (2012). Protecting the herd: A public health, economics, and legal argument for taxing parents who opt-out of mandatory childhood vaccinations. *Southern California Interdisciplinary Law Journal*, 21(2), 437–489.

Porter, D., and Porter, R. (1988). The politics of prevention: Anti-vaccinationism and public health in nineteenth-century England. *Medical History*, 32(03), 231–252.

PPPHW. (2015). About Global Handwashing Day. The Global Public-Private Partnership for Handwashing with Soap. Available at: www.globalhandwashing.org/source/ppphw

Resnik, D. (2004). Disclosing conflicts of interest to research subjects: An ethical and legal analysis. *Accountability in Research*, 11(2), 141–159.

Richins, C. (2011). Jacobson revisited: An argument for strict judicial scrutiny of compulsory vaccination. *Journal of Legal Medicine*, 32(4), 409–447.

Rodpothong, P., and Auewarakul, P. (2012). Viral evolution and transmission effectiveness. *World Journal of Virology*, 1(5), 131–134.

SAGE. (2014). *Report of the Sage Working Group on Vaccine Hesitancy*. Geneva: World Health Organization.

Saint-Victor, D. S., and Omer, S. B. (2013). Vaccine refusal and the endgame: Walking the last mile first. *Philosophical Transactions of the Royal Society of London B: Biological Sciences*, 368(1623), 20120148.

Sanofi. (2010). Sanofi-Aventis appoints Dr. Elias Zerhouni, president, global research and development. December 14. Available at: en.sanofi.com/Images/13798_20101214_nomination_en.pdf

*Sentaku* Magazine. (2014). Organizational flaws, collusive ties taking a toll on the WHO. *The Japan Times*. October 28. Available at: http://commentary/organizational-flaws-collusive-ties-taking-toll/#.Vx-vhDFf2Uk

Shah, S. (2011). How private companies are transforming the global public health agenda: A new era for the World Health Organization. Available at: www.foreigna ffairs.com/articles/136654/sonia-shah/how-private-companies-are-transforming-the-global-public-health (accessed April 27, 2016).

Silverman, R. D. (2003). No more kidding around: Restructuring non-medical child-hood immunization exemptions to ensure public health protection. *Annals of Health Law*, 12(2), 277–294.

Simpson, N., Lenton, S., and Randall, R. (1995). Parental refusal to have children immunised: Extent and reasons. *BMJ*, 310(6974), 225–227.

Smith, M. J., and Marshall, G. S. (2010). Navigating parental vaccine hesitancy. *Pediatric Annals*, 39(8), 476–482.

Smith, P. J., Chu, S. Y., and Barker, L. E. (2004). Children who have received no vaccines: Who are they and where do they live? *Pediatrics*, 114(1), 187–195.

Social Health and Family Affairs Committee (2010). The handling of the H1N1 pandemic: More transparency needed. *Doc. 12283* (Vol. 12). (Rapporteur: Mr. Paul Flynn). Strasbourg: Parliamentary Assembly of the Council of Europe.

Somerville, M., Kumaran, K., and Anderson, R. (2012). *Public Health and Epidemiology at a Glance*. Oxford: Wiley-Blackwell.

State of Israel Ministry of Health. (2013). Today a nationwide vaccination campaign against polio spread and carrying in Israel will start. August 18. Available at: www. health.gov.il/English/News_and_Events/Spokespersons_Messages

State of Israel Ministry of Health Haifa District Health Office. (2011). *A Summary of the Meeting of the Advisory Committee on Infectious Diseases and in the Ministry of Health Publications on Immunization, dated August 11, 2011 on the Presentation of Vaccines' Side Effects*. December 5. Haifa: State of Israel Ministry of Health Haifa District Health Office.

Stewardson, A., Allegranzi, B., Sax, H., Kilpatrick, C., and Pittet, D. (2011). Back to the future: Rising to the Semmelweis challenge in hand hygiene. *Future Microbiology*, 6(8), 855–876.

Stretch, R., Chambers, G., Whittaker, J., et al. (2008). Implementing a school-based HPV vaccination programme. *Nursing Times*, 104(48), 30–33.

Stuckler, D., King, L., Robinson, H., and McKee, M. (2008). WHO's budgetary allocations and burden of disease: A comparative analysis. *The Lancet*, 372(9649), 1563–1569.

Surowiecki, J. (2014). Ebolanomics. *The New Yorker*. August 25. Available at: www. newyorker.com/magazine/2014/08/25/ebolanomics

Task Force. (2015). Increasing appropriate vaccination: Monetary sanction policies. Available at: www.thecommunityguide.org/vaccines/MonetarySanctions.html (accessed April 26, 2016).

The State Comptroller and Ombudsman of Israel. (2014). *The Immunization Set for Children, Adults and Medical Staff. Annual Report 64c*. Available at: www.mevaker.

gov.il/he/Reports/Report_248/c51ffb79-e3a9-49b3-9654-8054462506ba/214-ver-4.pdf (In Hebrew) (accessed April 26, 2016).

U.S. Congress. (2015). H.R.2232 – Vaccinate All Children Act of 2015. May 1. Available at: www.congress.gov/bill/114th-congress/house-bill/2232/text.

U.S. Supreme Court. (1905). 197 U.S. 11. Henning Jacobson, plaintiff in error v. Commonwealth of Massachusetts, No. 70.

Velan, B., Boyko, V., Lerner-Geva, L., Ziv, A., Yagar, Y., and Kaplan, G. (2012). Individualism, acceptance and differentiation as attitude traits in the public's response to vaccination. *Human Vaccines and Immunotherapeutic*, 8(9), 1272–1282.

Vernon, J. G. (2003). Immunisation policy: From compliance to concordance? *British Journal of General Practice*, 53(490), 399–404.

Verweij, M., and Dawson, A. (2004). Ethical principles for collective immunisation programmes. *Vaccine*, 22(23–24), 3122–3126.

WHO. (2009). Hand hygiene: Why, how and when? Available at: www.who.int/gpsc/5may/Hand_Hygiene_Why_How_and_When_Brochure.pdf (accessed April 24, 2016).

WHO. (2015). Recommended composition of influenza virus vaccines for use in the 2015–2016 northern hemisphere influenza season. Available at: http://who.int/influenza/vaccines/virus/recommendations/201502_recommendation.pdf (accessed April 27, 2016).

Wolfe, R. M., and Sharp, L. K. (2002). Anti-vaccinationists past and present. *BMJ*, 325(7361), 430–432.

# 4 Strategies for Communicating Health Information and Risk

Health organizations face complex challenges in the 21st century, with the development of technology alongside the complexity of the world of epidemics. This chapter examines various strategies for risk communication used by health authorities to communicate epidemics and vaccinations in order to shape vaccine policies. Professional literature on risk management and risk communication emphasizes the importance of creating trust between the authorities and the public (Cvetkovich and Lofstedt, 1999; Earle and Cvetkovich, 1995; Lofstedt, 2005). Studies have found that when individuals who comprise the general public feel they have no control over a situation, trust in organizations is a key determinant in the public's reception of the risk management approach (Cvetkovich and Winter, 2002).

The social trust approach asserts that shared values between individuals and organizations to develop policy and make decisions is a key predictor of their trust in these organizations and in their risk management practices. Studies have found that individuals' level of openness rises when they believe that organizations and institutions hold similar salient values (Siegrist et al., 2000).

Furthermore, it has been found that there is a correlation between the level of trust and/or credibility people attribute to an organization and its communicator, and the extent to which they are willing to receive the organization's recommendations (McComas and Trumbo, 2001; Poortinga and Pidgeon, 2005; Siegrist et al., 2005). The more risk managers are perceived by the public as credible and confidence-inspiring, the more open and attentive the public will be to accept the health organizations' directives.

Trust is created by considering the needs and values of different publics, as well as the level of credibility of the organization. It would be expected that the authorities would adopt strategies that establish the credibility of the discourse. However, as Foucault (1980) argued, discourse is controlled by mechanisms that determine its limits: what one is allowed or is not allowed to discuss, where and how one should talk and to whom. Foucault emphasized that the mechanisms of power in society create a reality of truth and falsehoods within the scientific discourse – i.e., what is considered truth in the discourse, and what is defined as false. In the context of the discourse on epidemics, the desire to shape the truth, inasmuch as its power stems from mechanisms of control, refers to the use of force on those who hesitate or refuse to cooperate with guidelines.

The strategies exemplified in this chapter expose Foucault's claims, and raise the question of the ability of health organizations to create trust based on the credibility of the scientific discourse. This chapter will demonstrate how the strategy of truth and falsehood is transformed into myths, how scientific discourse is reduced to certainty, and how an epidemic turns into a "problem" that begs a solution. It will also demonstrate how the discourse preserves control mechanisms using statistical methodologies.

## Part 1 "Facts" versus "myths"

In their responses to concerns and fears raised by the public on topics related to vaccination and epidemics, leading health organizations such as the WHO and the CDC often use the term "myths" (CDC, 2015d; NHS, 2016; Public Health, 2016; WHO, 2016a). These organizations, as well as physicians' websites throughout the world, frame their answers in terms of "facts" versus "myths." In this context, myths are presented as misinformation and misconceptions believed by some members of the public. Those holding these beliefs are described as unaware that these myths are not true, biased, or based on false information. Spreading such myths leads to lack of compliance with the guidelines and recommendations of the health authorities (WHO, 2016b).

A myth is defined as a folktale that describes events that have significance or deep meaning for a particular community. In ancient times, gods and heroes were characters in myths, and modern myths contain metaphors and symbols of different types. The significance of a myth is that it generates a collective consciousness. A story can be considered a myth if it has the power to influence the behavior of those who are exposed to it (Segal, 2004). A myth has a complex relationship with the truth. On one hand, it must be persuasive. On the other hand, if it were true, it would be considered historical fact, not a myth.

Authorities' choice of using the word "myth" in relation to science is in fact a well-designed strategy, which can be examined in light of a vast theoretical literature on how myths are used to explain scientific phenomena.

Tylor (1920), an anthropologist who studied the evolution of science, argues that myth and religion helped premodern people to understand the world before modern science was developed. When science as we understand it today was developed, there was no longer any need for myth. Sir James George Frazer (2002), another social anthropologist, saw myth as practical science that helped humans control their environment by explaining the phenomena they observed or experienced. For Frazer, myth was a component of primitive religion, which served not only to explain natural phenomena, but also to ensure that they perpetuate. Both Taylor and Frazer considered a worldview steeped in myth to be one of the earliest steps towards scientific thinking.

Other researchers have indicated that we cannot distinguish between the mythopoetic approach (Frankfort et al., 1946) and a purely scientific approach. In light of this, they believed it would be misleading to contend that myths are unnecessary in modern times. They argued that myths continually shape human perception of reality – both ancient and modern.

Bultmann (1984) suggests approaching myths through a cultural, rather than a factual basis. Others, such as Karl Popper, have suggested that myth has a scientific purpose in modern times, and that addressing myths critically can promote scientific thinking. Popper argued:

> [S]cience must begin with myths, and with the criticism of myths; neither with the collection of observations, nor with the invention of experiments, but with the critical discussion of myths, and of magical techniques and practices.
>
> (2002, p. 66)

In this sense, Popper recognized the prevalence of uncertainty in scientific theories. In his view, theories cannot be decisively proven, and there should always be room for negating or contradicting them.

Malinowski argued that in ancient times, people did in fact approach the world from a scientific point of view. He writes:

> This brings us to the second question: Can we regard primitive knowledge, which, as we found, is both empirical and rational, as a rudimentary stage of science, or is it not at all related to it? If by science be understood a body of rules and conceptions, based on experience and derived from it by logical inference, embodied in material achievements and in a fixed form of tradition and carried on by some sort of social organization – then there is no doubt that even the lowest savage communities have the beginnings of science, however rudimentary.
>
> (Malinowski, 2014, p. 34)

Unlike Frazer and others, who viewed myth as a form of primitive scientific thinking, Malinowski believed that primitive man used science (what he called "primitive knowledge") in order to gain control over his surroundings, and when science did not work, he turned to magic. When magic was no longer useful, he turned to myth, not only to assert control over his surroundings, but also to deal with aspects that he could not control, such as disasters. According to Malinowski, myth explains what man cannot control.

These hypotheses about the function of myths in relation to scientific thought resonate in the present discussion of myth, in the context of risk perception regarding scientific phenomena, including epidemics. Experiments conducted by psychologists and risk communication researchers on risk perception and the decision-making process indicate that there is no clear distinction between "rational/science" and "intuitive/experiential." Such a distinction between logic and emotion is artificial, since people approach risk through a complex holistic perspective. Risk perception is influenced by personal, psychological, environmental, and cultural factors (Sandman, 2003; Slovic, 1999). Slovic, Finucane, Peters, and MacGregor (2004) have explored the association between the analytical and emotional aspects of risk perception, specifically the association between an analytical risk analysis and experience-based risk perception. The "analytical system" model was presented as a person's ability to analyze rules and norms, and calculate risks and opportunities, whereas the "experiential system" model was presented as intuitive, quick, automatic and partially subconscious. The studies in the literature assessing the public's risk perceptions deal alternately with analytical and experiential aspects.

We would thus argue that authorities' attempts to divide findings into "scientific facts" versus "myths" is likewise artificial. There is a continual interaction between feelings, thoughts, and experience, and laypeople and experts think in complex ways that are sometimes automatic, and "suffer" from biases in their perceptions (Kahneman et al., 1982).

Moreover, we would like to draw from Malinowski's line of thought that myths explain phenomena for which science does not offer satisfying or unequivocal explanations. When science incorporates uncertainty, people may tend to turn to myths in order to seek coherent and concrete explanations. Epidemics can be difficult to control or explain, and this is why the public might embrace myths, alongside scientific facts.

The authorities' strategy of choosing the word "myth" to convey the opposite of "fact" has several ramifications. First, it suggests that ideas contradicting the authorities' perspective are untrue. Second, it implies that authorities reflect the monolithic perspective of science, whereas all other perspectives reflect a mythopoetic approach that does not discern between objective and subjective perspectives. Third, it bespeaks a dichotomous distinction between experts and laypeople: whereas laypeople tend to be biased and lack understanding, authorities possess understanding and knowledge.

These claims lead to two main problems. The first concerns scientific content, and the second deals with how it is communicated. Regarding scientific content, there is a debate about issues connected to some vaccinations. The fact that every "doubt" is translated into a misconception undermines legitimate scientific debate. Moreover, every issue that involves elements of uncertainty becomes certain using the term "facts." This is exemplified by debates concerning how seasonal flu virus is presented. In recent years rigorous systematic reviews have raised questions as to the efficacy of influenza vaccines (Demicheli et al., 2014; Jefferson et al., 2010a; Jefferson et al., 2010b; Osterholm et al., 2012). For instance, Demicheli et al. (2014) and Jefferson et al. (2010b) found that influenza vaccines have a limited effect on reducing influenza symptoms. No evidence was found to indicate that these vaccines affect complications, such as pneumonia, or transmission. A systematic review conducted by Jefferson et al. (2010a) indicated that the available evidence regarding the safety, efficacy or effectiveness of influenza vaccines for people aged 65 years or older is of poor quality and provides no guidance. Nevertheless, on the CDC website (CDC, 2015d), only studies that support vaccination are cited – while studies presenting other perspectives are ignored. For example:

> [R]ecent study showed that flu vaccine reduced children's risk of flu-related pediatric intensive care unit (PICU) admission by 74% during flu seasons from 2010–2012. One study showed that flu vaccination was associated with a 71% reduction in flu-related hospitalizations among adults of all ages ... during the 2011–2012 flu season ...

The second problem raised by health authorities' use of the term "myths" is associated with the efficacy of risk communication (Bennett et al., 2010). Effective risk communication should be assessed not only by the technical aspect of communicating the risk, but rather, by how it takes into account the public's fears and concerns and deals with them, whether directly or indirectly. Effective risk communication addresses the public's various fears and concerns through dialogue. Transforming fears and concerns into "myth" or deeming them "false" undermines legitimate fears and concerns, and assumes that they are irrelevant falsehoods.

Research on risk perception has demonstrated that the lay public is not irrational, as is sometimes assumed when their response to risk is different from that expected by experts or public health recommendations. Rather, the public evaluates risks based on criteria and values not necessarily obvious to experts, but relevant to their everyday lives (Alaszewski, 2005). In this context, myths are based on discourse between peers and laypeople, and on experience accumulated in everyday life, notably through a practice that is social proof based on what can be regarded as practical evidence. The success of risk communication depends on the communicator's efforts to minimize the gap between the expert's risk assessments (evidence-based) and the public's perceptions (that can be derived from social proof), in order to create mutual feedback between experts and the public (Fischhoff, 2004). According to Sandman (1989), risk perception is comprised of hazard plus outrage. This means that other than the scientific aspect, feelings of outrage towards the risk must be considered. People associate high risk with issues towards which they have negative attitudes, regardless of the proved risk. The public's view of risk (as opposed to that of the experts) reflects not just the danger of the action (hazard), but also how they feel about the action and what emotions it produces (outrage). Lack of agreement between the experts' and the public's perception of hazard and outrage can lead to controversy. Like Sandman, Alhakami and Slovic (1994) found that affect influences decision-making. They found that the inverse relationship between perceived risk and perceived benefit of an activity is linked to the strength of positive or negative affect associated with that activity. This result implies that people's judgments are based not only on what they think about something, but also what they feel about it.

The disaccord between experts' point of view and that of the public cannot be allayed if authorities continue to see "outrage" or the "affect heuristic" as components that confound rational thinking. The gap between the experts and the public derives from distinct risk perceptions and different reactions. In reaction to the dissonance between the perspectives of the authorities and that of the public, authorities want the public to understand that their perspective must be transformed. Such an attitude does not mitigate the gap. Moreover, the very fact that the intuitive or emotional component is framed as "mythic" or as "false" perpetuates the distance between the experts and the public, rather than mitigating the gap. Dialogue between the public and experts should be based on emotional and cognitive components, as well as on the public's collective memory.

Several studies confirm the authorities' failure in using the strategy of "Facts" versus "Myths." For example, despite efforts by the Centers for Disease Control and Prevention (CDC, 2015a) to undermine vaccination myths and despite almost universal support for vaccinations among healthcare providers, compliance with vaccination against seasonal flu remained low (CDC, 2015e).

In two studies on public perception of the MMR vaccine and the seasonal flu vaccine (Nyhan and Reifler, 2015; Nyhan et al., 2014), they presented parents with pro-vaccine information from the CDC website. However, these pro-vaccine messages failed to improve parents' attitudes toward vaccination. In fact, these studies reported a "backfire effect": vaccine skeptics formed even stronger negative opinions about vaccinations after being given information intended to undermine the supposed connection between vaccinations and autism. They concluded:

> Future research should continue to explore the causal relationship between vaccine misperceptions and vaccine hesitancy. If misperceptions cause vaccine hesitancy, then debunking those myths should increase willingness to vaccinate. But if misperceptions are the expression of a more generalized antipathy toward vaccines, then addressing these myths piecemeal is unlikely to be effective. A more comprehensive strategy is likely to be required.
>
> (Nyhan and Reifler, 2015, p. 463)

Along similar lines, Horne, Powell, Hummel, and Holyoak (2015) also explored the CDC's strategy of debunking myths. They showed that not only are these strategies ineffective, but that they intensify and increase opposition. The results of their study reveal the effectiveness of presenting facts to change attitudes: convincing parents that the probability of disease contraction is high if they do not vaccinate their children and that the consequences of getting these illnesses can be severe. This approach is analogous to that taken by researchers who have effectively corrected participants' erroneous beliefs, not by refuting incorrect elements of these beliefs, but rather by replacing those elements with new information. They successfully countered people's anti-vaccination attitudes by making them appreciate the consequences of failing to vaccinate their children (using information provided by the CDC). This intervention outperformed another that aimed to undermine widespread vaccination myths.

However, this point of view is countered by Graves (2015), who contends that arguing the facts does not help. In fact, it might even worsen the situation. According to his article, people will only accept evidence that fits their pre-existing views. In addition, he argues that authorities do not resort to empathy, preferring to censure the parents who refuse or hesitate – a practice that has been found to be ineffective. Graves suggests creating narratives to which people can relate and that are relevant to their lives, rather than refuting their feelings.

This discussion exposes how health authorities address the issue of sharing facts with the public. It demonstrates that they resort to the strategy of subverting myths. The problem is that defining issues in such terms creates an impasse between the experts and the public and leaves no room for two-way communication.

Authorities should consider different framings. Instead of using the frame of "facts" versus "myths," they might want to consider the most effective way to conduct a debate with the (often skeptical) public. Drawing from the critical approach of Karl Popper, they might ask: how can we convey information that includes scientific doubt and uncertainty? In shaping this question, they might want to avoid a perspective that supports a dichotomous division into "facts" (put forward by the authorities) and "myths" (believed by the public that does not comply with the authorities). They should attempt to conduct this scientific debate by addressing controversial matters and issues of uncertainty directly and honestly.

## Part 2 Casting uncertainty in certain terms

In the changing and unpredictable world of epidemics, one of the most significant challenges faced by health organizations is decision-making in conditions of uncertainty. It is impossible to predict the trajectory of epidemics, and even viruses considered obsolete can appear in mutated forms, that are immune to vaccinations used previously, and therefore call for new strategies. Conditions of uncertainty raise difficult questions with regard to ethics, communication, and management. Despite this, the organizations tend to simplify out of the belief that the public seeks clear answers, and also in order to promote their policies.

Uncertainty refers to any situation in which the consequences are unknown – whether due to inadequate data (Einhorn and Hogwarth, 1985), or because of incomplete scientific understanding or an indeterminate chain of causality (Wynne, 1992). This, in turn, leads to vagueness from the decision-makers' point of view (Wallsten, 1990). Risk scholars have stressed that dealing with uncertain risks is an important challenge in risk management and assessment (Fox, 2009; Lofstedt, 2005; Nowotny et al., 2001; Ravetz, 2001; Renn, 2006; Wynne, 1992, 1995).

Increasingly, researchers argue that uncertainty and risk are not mutually distinguishable as easily as was assumed by the positivistic risk paradigm (Nowotny et al., 2001; Renn and Walker, 2008; van Asselt and Vos, 2006, 2008). Risk has been described as referring "objectively to the circumstances of the physical world" (Shrader-Frechette, 1996; Thompson and Dean, 1996). In contrast, according to constructivists, it is only relevant to talk about risk in particular settings (Adams, 1995; Hilgartner, 1992). Constructivists view risk management and assessment as inseparable, with value differences at the core. For example, van Asselt and Vos (2008, p. 281) argue that, "Uncertain risks need to be sharply distinguished from traditional, simple risks which can be calculated by means of statistics." According to Klinke and Renn, constructivists view risk and risk assessments to "constitute mental constructions that can be checked at best against standards of consistency, cohesion and internal conventions of logical deduction" (Klinke and Renn, 2002, p. 1073).

Scholars have acknowledged that uncertainty is a salient feature of societal debates on new technologies, an inevitable by-product or "side effect" of innovation (Fox, 2009; Nowotny et al., 2001).

### *Declaring an epidemic in conditions of uncertainty: Case studies*

In declaring an epidemic, conditions of uncertainty may lead to two opposing reactions – either to hesitation or to declaring an epidemic prematurely. We analyzed health organizations' declarations of an epidemic in two instances: that of the H1N1 outbreak in 2009, and the recent Ebola epidemic. In both situations, we found that the declarations did not acknowledge uncertainty.

The purpose of the first study was to examine the communication that took place between two central health authorities – the World Health Organization (WHO) and the Centers for Disease Control and Prevention (CDC), and the media, during the 2009 outbreak of the H1N1 influenza virus. The virtual press briefings held by both organizations during the outbreak and published by them provided an opportunity to examine the media's response during the outbreak.

Regarding H1N1, we analyzed 2009 press releases from the WHO CDC. We examined 26 transcripts of virtual press conferences held by the WHO that took place between May 5, 2009 and August 10, 2010, as well as 53 transcripts of virtual press conferences held by the CDC that took place between April 23, 2009 and March 29, 2010. The transcripts documented the virtual meetings between the WHO and CDC representatives, and health journalists from media outlets around the world.

Notwithstanding considerable uncertainty and vagueness expressed in their responses regarding the disease, both WHO and CDC representatives framed the outbreak as a pandemic long before a pandemic was actually declared. All along, they gave the impression that the virus was dangerous and even lethal, and they stressed that although data suggested that the disease was mild, the situation could change any minute. They used the 1918 Influenza Pandemic as a precedent for such a situation.

> *The WHO was accused of hyping the pandemic* and I'm wondering whether this might pose problems for you in the future if and when a new pandemic arises?
>
> (WHO, 2010, p. 7)

> I just wanted to ask Dr. Chan, are you still convinced that you made the right call in June of 2009 to declare the pandemic, *in view of the heavy criticism that followed?*
>
> (WHO, 2010, p. 2)

Whereas the 2009 H1N1 outbreak was an example of the phenomenon of "hyping the disease," we found that a different phenomenon occurred when the Ebola crisis erupted. The WHO did not rush to declare an epidemic, but instead used the term "outbreak." This wording framed the crisis in different terms and shaped the WHO's global approach.

The *Report of the Ebola Interim Assessment Panel* revealed a delay in declaring a public health emergency of international concern (Panel of Independent Experts, 2015). The report acknowledges political and economic reasons for the delay:

> Delay in the declaration of a PHEIC stemmed from: concerns about challenging governments; understandable worries about economic and trade implications for the countries affected; the fact that WHO had been previously criticized for declaring a PHEIC for pandemic influenza H1N1; and lack of data resulting from conflicting definitions of cases and the unwillingness of various actors to share data for aggregation.
>
> (Panel of Independent Experts, 2015, p. 13)

Preferring the term "outbreak" over "epidemic" affected how the disease was conceptualized, thereby influencing the risk signature. The terms the authorities employed to communicate the risk of Ebola, either as a "mere" outbreak or as a more serious epidemic, influenced the public's response, attitudes and behaviors (Gesser-Edelsburg et al., 2016). Our sample included online websites of three leading newspapers from three different countries: *The New York Times* (the USA), *Daily Mail* (the UK) and *Ynet* (Israel). *The New York Times* is the second largest newspaper in circulation in the USA (Associated Press, 2013); *Daily Mail* is the most read newspaper brand in the UK (Ponsford, 2016), and *Ynet* has a 36.4% share of the Israeli market according to a TGI survey (Wertheim, 2014). We gathered 582 articles: 80 articles from *The New York Times*, 444 from the *Daily Mail*, and 58 articles from *Ynet*. We analyzed all of the online articles that reported on the Ebola disease from each newspaper's website. The span of the articles was from March 23, 2014, the date on which the WHO declared an outbreak of the Ebola disease, to September 30, 2014, when the first case of Ebola was reported in the United States.

In light of this surge, the ongoing Ebola crisis should be defined in terms of an epidemic. This is because, according to the literature, an outbreak is a sudden rise in the occurrence (number of cases) of a disease (Aronson and Shope, 2008), whereas an epidemic is the occurrence of more cases of a disease than is anticipated in a community or region during a given period in light of previous experience. Although each of these terms has been delineated, experts still mull over which terms to use in light of the emphases associated with each term. The terms outbreak and epidemic are used interchangeably and sometimes together by many epidemiologists and in the professional literature (CDC, 2012g; Green et al., 2002; Macera et al., 2013). Each term entails different political and policy implications, as well as their significance for the public.

Leading health organizations, such as the WHO and the CDC, tended to classify Ebola as an "outbreak." For example, a news release published on the WHO website on September 19, 2014, dubbed the current Ebola epidemic an "ongoing outbreak." Similarly, one CDC website headline was "2014 Ebola Outbreak in West Africa." By contrast, in his speech on September 16, 2014 at the CDC, American President Barack Obama characterized Ebola as an "epidemic." Although in later speeches, Obama attempted to reassure the public regarding the crisis, behind the scenes he was expressed concern about the escalating danger, and went so far as to criticize the CDC for its response as being "not tight."

It is not surprising that the term "outbreak" was most prevalent in the articles that preceded Obama's speech. Although in general, the terms "outbreak" and "epidemic" are used interchangeably, and sometimes together by many epidemiologists and in the professional literature (CDC, 2012g; Green et al., 2002; Macera et al., 2013), in the case of the current Ebola crisis, the term "outbreak" has been the one leading health authorities consistently employed. It is possible the authorities' choice to continue using the term "outbreak" stemmed from their previous experience with declaring diseases "epidemics" – the WHO was castigated for misrepresenting the threat of the H1N1 crisis, claiming it was more serious that it actually was (Social Health and Family Affairs Committee, 2010). In addition, researchers tend to assume that the general population perceives the term "epidemic" somewhat differently from that intended by epidemiologists. According to the CDC, the public is more likely to think that epidemic implies a crisis situation (CDC, 2012g), and indeed, the popular literature uses the term "epidemic" to indicate an outbreak associated with greater risk and greater danger to the public and afflicting a large number of victims (Green et al., 2002). In light of this, health authorities may have chosen the term "outbreak" as a precaution to allay public fears.

According to Frewer et al. (2003), experts tend to believe that the public is unable to conceptualize uncertainties associated with risk management processes, and that providing it with information about uncertainty might generate panic and confusion and increase distrust in science and scientific institutions. Yet, this belief has been shown to be inaccurate. Studies have indicated that in situations of risk, especially risks that involve uncertainty, the public wants full transparency of information. Transparent communication does not provoke negative reactions among the public, but, rather, helps reduce negative feelings, and increases the public's respect for the risk-assessing agency (De Vocht et al., 2016; Lofstedt, 2006; Palenchar and Heath, 2002; Slovic, 1991, 1995). Despite this, in practice, the organizations prefer to adopt other tactics. In what follows, we discuss some of them.

### *Lack of transparency in situations of uncertainty*

Situations of uncertainty can cause organizations to adopt what is known as "strategic ambiguity," using ambiguity purposefully to accomplish particular goals (Eisenberg, 1984). Ambiguity is sometimes used by governments and organizations to build internal and/or external organizational credibility among people who do not know how to act in the absence of a clear disconfirming message.

Strategic ambiguity can promote economic, political, organizational, or diplomatic interests. Sometimes this strategy involves the manipulative use of facts and providing an interpretation that corresponds with the communicator's policy and interest. It may be used to avoid guilt and personal responsibility (Ulmer and Sellnow, 1997). Strategic ambiguity may be employed to express ongoing ambiguity, like Israel's policy of nuclear ambiguity (Baliga and Sjöström, 2008) or it can be used during a specific crisis. In such a case, strategic ambiguity can be expressed by the use of vague language. It can also be conveyed by language that rationalizes and justifies certain actions. Usually strategic ambiguity employs selective information, sometimes distorting facts. Strategic ambiguity enables the communicator to reframe reality. In the context of risk communication, it may treat the risk level differently from the public while trying to persuade the public to accept the communicator's point of view.

A prominent example of the use of strategic ambiguity is the polio outbreak in Israel. In February 2013, Israel's Health Ministry reported that wild poliovirus type 1 (WPV1) had been detected in environmental sewage samples from southern and central Israel. WPV1 was subsequently isolated in stool samples from 42 carriers (4.4% of the sampled population) tested in area of WPV1 circulation (Ministry of Health Israel, 2013a). All viruses were detected in sewage and random stool samples only, and no clinical cases of paralytic polio were reported (Ministry of Health Israel, 2013a, 2013b, 2013e, 2013f, 2013g). After the latest detection of WPV1, the Health Ministry launched a supplementary campaign in early August 2013, immunizing children under age 10 (already protected by IPV) with a bivalent OPV vaccine (OPV 1 and 3) (Ministry of Health Israel, 2013c).

In order to expose the barriers that inhibited parental compliance with OPV vaccination for their children, we conducted a survey during the polio outbreak in Israel, and also analyzed readers' comments and Facebook discussions (Gesser-Edelsburg, Shir-Raz, and Green, 2016). Our findings indicate that some parents who normally give their children routine vaccinations decided against the OPV for diverse reasons. Some parents vaccinated their children because they actually misunderstood the reason for vaccinating. They vaccinated because they understood that OPV was to protect their own children, whereas it was intended for overall societal well-being.

The research findings revealed that the public felt it was being given ambiguous explanations and vague answers:

> The difficulty in making the decision stems from the ambiguity surrounding basic questions such as exactly who needs to be vaccinated, who is at risk from the vaccine, who has to get it and who is advised not to, but it comes mainly from parents' inability to understand the real reason for the vaccines.
>
> (Shafran-Gittelman, 2013)

To a certain extent, the Health Ministry intended to convey an ambiguous message. The campaign, called "Two Drops," was promoted by the slogan: "Just two drops will protect the family from the polio threat." This led some parents to understand that the vaccination was intended to protect their own children.

Sometimes organizations use "cover-up communication," a term coined by Gesser-Edelsburg and Zemach (2012). Unlike the strategy of ambiguous communication, in this situation, the organization accepts the risk perceptions of the public. The organization uses clear and coherent language on a frequent basis to update the public with information based on unbiased data. However, when organizations avoid and deflect attempts to answer the question "why?" or to address what caused a particular disaster, this is "cover-up risk communication." This involves credible, inclusive, and transparent crisis communication. It entails providing the public with complete information and unbiased data, emphasizing operative actions occurring in the present; and ways of managing and preventing the risk in the future, while avoiding serious discussion of antecedents of the crisis, in order to avoid guilt and personal responsibility. Both strategies, strategic ambiguity and cover-up risk communication, attempt to cover up a failure and avoid personal responsibility. In each strategy, the risk is communicated differently. Whereas the language of strategic ambiguity is neither clear nor transparent and its point of departure is a denial of the audience's perception of reality (its perception of the risk level), cover-up risk communication is outwardly clear and transparent, shares the audience's risk perception, and communicates with it.

### The science is clear!

Following the 2015 "Disneyland Measles Outbreak," former U.S. Secretary of State and future Democratic presidential candidate Hillary Clinton critiqued several likely Republican rivals who argued that parents should be able to choose how their children are vaccinated. In a Tweet, Clinton commented: "The science is clear: The earth is round, the sky is blue, and vaccines work" (Clinton, 2015). This tweet exemplifies how authorities claim ownership of science, labeling anyone who does not comply with their guidelines and recommendations as extremist or even delusional.

The literature indicates that in situations of uncertainty, policy makers do not always provide full information and instead, use science to frame uncertainty in terms of absolute certainty. Van Asselt and Vos (2008, p. 281) term such situations the "uncertainty paradox." This refers to situations where uncertainty is acknowledged, but the role of science is framed as providing certainty. Analyses of actual cases of EU risk regulation conducted by van Asselt and Vos (2005, 2006) and (Fox, 2009) demonstrate that the uncertainty paradox leads to unintelligible policy making processes. Moreover, they argue that sometimes, uncertainty is not even acknowledged (Fox, 2009). They use the term "uncertainty intolerance," borrowed from psychology, to describe such situations. In psychology, the term "uncertainty intolerance" is used to refer to people who cannot accept that something negative might happen, regardless of the chances (Vlaeyen, 2008). A similar term used in risk perception literature is "risk aversive" (Slovic, 1991). Van Asselt and Vos (2008, p. 281) explain that unlike "risk aversive," uncertainty intolerance in the context of policy-making refers to situations in which institutions and organizations do not acknowledge the uncertainty and are *unwilling* to demand and produce information on uncertainty. Instead of systematically investigating the uncertainty, they choose to regard it as irrelevant, or simply ignore it. In his analysis, Fox (2009) found that in some cases, even when some stakeholders do acknowledge the uncertainty and provide uncertainty information, when a dominant or influential stakeholder who is intolerant of uncertainty enters the scene, they can impose uncertainty intolerance. Researchers argue that this may result in unintelligible risk regulation. To establish regulation, Health Ministry officials tend not to use the language of risk communication. Rather than expressing clear and balanced information, incorporating diverging points of view and concerns of different subpopulations, they chose to promote the uncertainty in certain terms. Van Asselt and Vos (2008) and van Asselt, Vos, and Rooijackers (2009) emphasize these strategies in the various cases of risk regulation at the European level. Although uncertainty is acknowledged and some actors express uncertainty tolerance, crucial actors demand certainty at the same time.

Similarly, a study conducted in the UK (Christley et al., 2013) found that many models commissioned by governments during outbreaks provide only cursory reference to the uncertainties entailed by the information, data or parameters used. The researchers analyzed scientific papers, interviews, policies, reports and outcomes of infectious disease outbreaks in the UK, and concluded that while the models were uncertain, many still informed action. Limitations and uncertainties were sometimes not addressed.

The same phenomenon is also revealed in a case study we conducted during the Ebola epidemic, based on the Hickox quarantine incident. On October 23, 2014, Kaci Hickox, a nurse who returned from treating Ebola patients in Sierra Leone, was quarantined at a New Jersey hospital (Gesser-Edelsburg and Shir-Raz, 2015). The study focused on newspaper coverage of the case and readers' comments on newspaper articles. We examined how the media and the public perceived the precautionary measures taken by authorities, in light of the ongoing crisis whose spread was uncertain. One of the findings that emerged from this study indicated that the U.S. public health establishment proclaimed Ebola absolutism, referring to scientific evidence against Ebola quarantines as "'the science' instead of just 'science',", and thus attacking the pro-quarantine opinion with which they disagreed, as "unscientific."

Some readers' comments exposed the problem with conveying certainty about an issue that actually entails uncertainty. The following response by J. Andrew addresses the debate about virus transmission:

> While the opponents widely used "the science" to back to their arguments, supporters stressed that science is a field in which uncertainty is "built-in", and that there are no "100% truths" in it: 'Everyone keeps talking about the "science" and respect for the "science", but it's worth pointing out that the science is very uncertain.
>
> (*The New York Times*, October 31, 2014)

Given that Ebola transmission is still characterized by uncertainty, quarantine supporters tended to reinforce their claims with scientific evidence. A prominent claim from the public concerned the fact that authorities who opposed quarantine did not raise issues of uncertainty. This criticism reinforces the claims of van Asselt and Vos (2008), who discuss the uncertainty paradox in conditions wherein uncertainty is acknowledged, but the role of science is framed as providing certainty.

Sandman and Lanard (2011) emphasize the need to "proclaim uncertainty," advising authorities to share tentative information if that is all they have. Similarly, regarding Ebola, Rosenbaum (2015) claims that although health authorities cannot know everything, they should share information.

Furthermore, treating the public as ignorant of science and refraining from providing full transparency of information might backfire at the authorities. As Wynne (2001) warns, institutional science's attempts to exaggerate its intellectual control and use knowledge as justification of policy commitments, while ignoring its limits, only alienates the public and increases its mistrust.

The campaign launched by the Israeli Health Ministry during the 2013 polio crisis (discussed above) also demonstrates how certain terms were used in communication with the public despite a fundamental uncertainty. The former CEO of the Israeli Health Ministry maintained that the vaccination had "zero side effects." He said this in the context of the ministry's efforts to convince parents to vaccinate children already vaccinated with the IPV vaccine with a bivalent OPV vaccine (OPV 1 and 3). They chose to frame it in exclusively positive and popular (unscientific) terms.

These situations lead us to argue that the term "uncertainty intolerance" is an understatement, because sometimes health organizations conduct campaigns that disregard or reject all studies that do not support the official representative's agenda, claiming that they do not uphold professional standards. Policy makers often criticize laypeople, such as bloggers on the social networks, for sharing only partial information with the public on topics that concern public health, accusing them of spreading misleading information and misconceptions. We argue that the policy makers themselves do exactly this, carrying out what they accuse laypeople of doing. They share only partial, biased information in order to support their case, and convey information in terms that misrepresent the actual situation. We propose calling such a phenomenon "uncertainty bias," in which the policy makers frame uncertainty in biased terms.

One example of when this bias becomes conspicuous is when it is stated that there is a consensus on a particular topic, when in fact, there is no consensus and opinions are divided. This can lead policy makers to make decisions based on situations that seem clear-cut, when in fact understanding the controversy might have led them to other conclusions. In addition, this has consequences for the public. The public's decisions are affected by framing, and, as such, if the public thinks that there is certainty, this understanding will guide its actions.

## Part 3 The epidemic narrative

"A vicious enemy has evaded our country." This dramatic statement is how Israel's former Health Minister, Yael German, open her announcement on the national vaccination campaign launched in 2013, following the detection of the polio virus in Israeli sewage (German, 2013; Kaliner et al., 2015; Matzliah, 2013). Using her Facebook feed, as well as interviews on television and other media outlets, German described the enemy, "It is smart and sly, it operates under the radar, it cannot be seen but it works tirelessly, penetrating every possible body and proliferating." She stated, "We are now in a war to defeat it and prevent the disease." Such dramatic descriptions of infectious disease outbreaks as a vicious and cunning enemy are part of a prevalent strategy used by health organizations and officials to frame outbreaks and vaccines – a strategy which we have dubbed "the epidemic narrative."

Matheson (2008) describes how, in order to promote their drugs and influence policy-making through the construction of scientific and medical knowledge, pharmaceutical companies create "a drug narrative" – a story or script "in which 'problems' arise and are 'solved' by drugs" (Matheson, 2008, p. 355). This story is used in order to frame the information about the drug, and includes "environmental messages" about the disease (i.e., claims about the area of medicine in which the drug is marketed – frequently identifying "unmet needs"). Contrastingly, it also includes specific "product messages" (i.e., claims about the drug – including claims that it meets "unmet needs").

Like every narrative, the drug narrative built by the pharma industries is based on myths. It is constructed like the classic narrative of villains and heroes (Shir-Raz, 2014). Villains and heroes are two of the fundamental myths, which, according to Jack Lule (2001), are commonly used in journalistic texts. Lule believes that each society is based on several fundamental myths, which take the form of archetypes. In modern society, he suggests, the journalists play the role of the ancient storytellers. News stories are based on the same archetypes, and also play the same role, which is to maintain social order. Similarly, it was found that press releases delivered to health journalists by pharmaceutical companies are based on two fundamental myths – the "villain" and the "hero" (Shir-Raz, 2014). While diseases are portrayed in terms of a "villain," plotting to destroy humanity, drugs are presented as the ultimate "hero," coming to the rescue of humankind. Some 42.9% of 1,465 press releases delivered by pharmaceutical companies to health journalists in Israel from 1 January 2003 to 30 December 2012 used such myths. Thus, what Matheson (2008) calls "the problem" is portrayed as a "villain" in the pharma's narrative, and the "solution" is "the hero." Since, as Lule (2001) found, employing myths is common journalistic practice, by employing the same myths, the pharmaceutical companies and their PR consultants ensure that their stories get published (Shir-Raz, 2014).

Yet, the pharma industries are not alone in using this strategy to promote their messages. The current chapter will demonstrate how health organizations also tend to adopt the same strategy, including its questionable tactics, to frame outbreaks and promote vaccination. This framing is built using the same two mythical characters – the villain and the hero.

### Depicting the vicious enemy: the outbreak

The first player to appear in the pharma's plot is the "villain." Presenting the villain myth – or what Matheson (2008) calls "the problem," serves to build broad public awareness of various diseases and brand them. For this purpose, as scholars have indicated, drug companies often employ intimidation tactics (Arnst, 2006; Moynihan and Cassels, 2005; Parsons, 2007). According to Parsons (2007), these include emotional appeal, or in Aristotle's terms – the "pathos" approach. The emotional appeal relies largely on an overly dramatic rhetoric, describing the disease not "just" as a disease, but as a devious and cruel enemy – "a vicious killer," a "silent murderer," "a dangerous enemy."

In contrast, the emotional rhetoric is reinforced by extensive use of what can be seen as cognitive appeal, or in Aristotle's terms, the "logos" approach: using statistics and data from surveys and polls or citing "experts' estimations" or "predictions" to describe diseases prevalence and the risk, suffering, and problems associated with them. Yet, the statistics used are selective, intended to exaggerate the prevalence of the disease and the risks and suffering it entails (Shir-Raz, 2014). Employing statistics and numbers manufactures a "quantification rhetoric," which, according to Petersen and Lupton (1996, p. 38), "tends to suggest the figures used are not subject to doubt or uncertainty." The power of quantification is not that it indicates an objective measurement of certain aspects of the real world, but that by turning those aspects into numbers provides a sense of certainty, which is very persuasive (Dew, 2012). Thus, the use of "quantification rhetoric" to describe the disease, especially when coupled with verbal rhetoric, serves to increase the drama and help maintain the villain myth and to manufacture intimidation and fear.

In a similar manner, health organizations and officials often portray outbreaks as a vicious enemy, using the same intimidation tactics to promote vaccination. A prominent example is the portrayal of measles outbreaks. For instance, Peter Strebel from the Department of Immunization, Vaccines and Biologicals in WHO's Geneva headquarters, states: "This disease is a tough enemy. Too many countries at risk of measles epidemics don't realise how tough it is" (Maurice, 2015). In a press conference marking the 50th Anniversary of the Measles Vaccine (CDC, 2013b), Strebel states again that "despite this progress, measles remains a formidable enemy." Similarly, following the 2015 measles outbreak in California, Tom Frieden, the Director of the Centers for Disease Control and Prevention, stated: "Measles is a personal enemy of mine" (Frieden, 2015).

In some cases, the dramatic rhetoric is accompanied by visuals, thereby reinforcing the emotional appeal and increasing fear. Dew (1999) describes how during the 1997 measles outbreak in New Zealand, the Ministry of Health ran an advertisement campaign in newspapers and on television, using powerful imagery to frighten parents into vaccinating children. "The viewer was subjected to images of cemeteries and crucifixes passing across the screen, followed by a pulsating brain. Slowly, an outline of a young boy emerged with the message 'don't join the dots'" (Dew, 1999, p. 388). This emotional appeal was supported by a cognitive appeal, using "quantification rhetoric," as the message in the advertisements for measles vaccine in the printed media presented scary quantitative estimates of the numbers of complications and deaths:

> We estimate that 45,000 New Zealand children will be hit by the Measles epidemic this year. Of these, four thousand will have ear infections, pneumonia or diarrhoea. Approximately nine hundred will be hospitalized. Thirty will suffer brain inflammation. Up to nine will be left with permanent brain damage. At least four will die. You have a choice. Talk to your doctor about free immunization and remove the risk of Measles forever. Or pray your child doesn't join the dots. Measles. It's not a pretty picture.
>
> (Dew, 1999, p. 388)

These terrifying predictions are exacerbated by the fact that the 1997 outbreak in New Zealand turned out to be minor. The actual number of cases of measles reported was 1,200, and not a single child died (Dew, 1999).

Nevertheless, the mixture of quantification rhetoric and the overly dramatic verbal rhetoric forged a clear message: "Have your child vaccinated, or risk their death from the brain-pulsating condition of encephalitis" (Dew, 1999, p. 388).

Another striking example of the employment of intimidation tactics to promote vaccination is the way human papilloma virus (HPV) is described by health authorities and experts. Like measles, HPV is also depicted as a cruel and cunning enemy, plotting its attack silently in the shadows. In her book *Cervical Cancer*, Spencer (2007) entitles the fourth chapter, which focuses on HPV, "Public Enemy Number 1: Human Papillomavirus." Similarly, the authors of scientific articles focusing on HPV have chosen titles such as "Human Papillomavirus: A Catalyst to a Killer" (Richman, 2005), and "The invisible enemy – how human papillomaviruses avoid recognition and clearance by the host immune system" (Grabowska and Riemer, 2012). "HPV remains a silent killer because people don't know about it," states McCafferty (2006), the editor of *ADVANCE for Nurses*.

Alongside those depictions of the virus, quantification rhetoric is often used. For instance, the CDC website states: "HPV is a very common virus; nearly 80 million people – about one in four – are currently infected in the United States" (CDC, 2015f). The NIH website, citing the CDC, estimates that "more than 90 percent and 80 percent, respectively, of sexually active men and women will be infected with at least one type of HPV at some point in their lives" (NIH, 2015).

In addition, data on cervical cancer are presented by focusing on global statistics. For example, at an Israeli parliament meeting in 2007 on the accelerated approval of the HPV vaccine, Professor Jacob Bornstein, President of the International Society for the Study of Vulvovaginal Disease, and then-head of the national Society for Cervical Cancer and head of obstetrics in Galilee Medical Center-Nahariya, explained: "Cervical cancer is the second most common cause of death in women worldwide, and the first most common in developing countries, and those numbers explain why so much effort and money were invested to find a vaccine" (The Committee for the Advancement of Women's Status, 2007).

Yet, these overly dramatic depictions and statistics are often highlighted while omitting other vital information. First, most of HPV infections are temporary and clear spontaneously, without progressing to cervical cancer (Goldstein et al., 2009; Hathaway, 2012; National Advisory Committee on Immunization, 2007; Schiffman and Kjaer, 2003). In fact, the most important predictor of cervical cancer is that persistent infections do not go away. Only a small number of these infections eventually develop into cervical cancer (Schiffman and Kjaer, 2003). Second, while it might be true that, globally, cervical cancer is the second most common cancer and the second leading cause of cancer mortality in women, 80–85% of cervical cancer cases and more than 85% of the deaths occur in developing countries (Jemal et al. 2010; Parkin, 2006; WHO, 2015). In western countries, it is actually relatively rare (Lowy, 2011). Furthermore, as Connell and Hunt (2010) argue, there has been no significant increase in the incidence of cervical cancer. In fact, pap tests are a reliable method for detecting cervical diseases and their extensive use has resulted in an 80% reduction in deaths from cervical cancer in western countries. Thus, choosing to focus on global statistics instead of on those relevant to western countries creates an impression that the prevalence of the disease is much higher than it really is.

It is interesting to note that, as an Israeli study found, the same overly dramatic rhetoric and selective statistics noted above were used by MSD Pharmaceutical, a subsidiary of Merck and Co – the manufacturer of Gardasil – to promote the vaccine's approval and funding in Israel in 2007–2012. By choosing to adopt this rhetoric and to cite selective statistics, health organizations and officials have in fact adopted the framing created by the industry.

Moreover, the organizations have adopted the framing chosen by the pharma, relating to the vaccine as a "cervical cancer vaccine," instead of an "HPV vaccine." A WHO communication guide for countries about introducing the HPV vaccine (WHO, 2013a), advises: "In general, countries refer to the HPV vaccine as a '*cancer vaccine*', rather than a vaccine against a sexually transmitted infection." According to the document's authors, "This is sensible for many reasons. For one, people will know and fear cancer more than HPV (which they may have never heard about). If the perceived benefit is to prevent a cancer, the vaccine will probably pique more interest and demand" (WHO, 2013a, p. 39).

According to Connell and Hunt (2010), the fact that this link to cervical cancer is at the center of HPV vaccination campaigns is not surprising. They argue, "It is significant that the 'evil' that the HPV project is directed against is a cancer, today's most dreaded disease" (Connell and Hunt, 2010, p. 67). As a villain, there is no doubt that cancer is much more intimidating than a virus, and thus provides a much more powerful motivation for compliance.

A third example of adopting intimidation tactics to promote vaccination, which has unfortunately become increasingly prominent over the past two decades, is seasonal influenza. Analyzing how influenza vaccination is promoted by the CDC, Doshi (2013) argues that it involves "marketing influenza as a threat of great proportions." While the CDC website explains: "Flu seasons are unpredictable and can be severe," and estimates a death toll of "3000 to a high of about 49 000 people" in the USA, Doshi indicates a far less volatile and frightening picture of influenza when considering that in the mid-20th century, mortality rates associated with influenza declined sharply. This decline, he claims, is a source of greater optimism when added to the fact that it happened before "the great expansion of vaccination campaigns in the 2000s, and despite three so-called 'pandemics'." The significant change brought about by these campaigns stemmed from expanding the perception of who is "at risk" – i.e., the transition from targeting an older segment of the population to targeting the general population. This transition is exemplified not only on the CDC website, but also by many other marketing tools, such as YouTube videos and social media. For instance, an article posted on the social media through Thunderclap, a crowdspeaking platform that empowers and boosts social networks, presents a smiling family, including grandparents, parents and three children. It warns that "Influenza (flu) is a serious disease that can lead to hospitalization and sometimes even death … Even healthy people can get very sick from the flu and spread it to others." The post concludes: "Everyone 6 months and older should get an annual flu vaccine" (CDC and NFID, 2015).

One could argue that the authorities do not intend to generate fear. Rather, they believe these conjectures and are concerned about their implications. Yet, a CDC PowerPoint presentation entitled "Planning for the 2004–05 Influenza Vaccination Season: A Communication Situation Analysis," tells a different story. The presentation, prepared by Glen Nowak, then-CDC Acting Director of Media Relations, and Associate Director for Communications at the NIP, includes a "Seven-Step Recipe for Generating Interest in, and Demand for, Flu (or any other) Vaccination" (Nowak, 2004). Generating demand for vaccines, Nowak explains in the presentation, "requires creating concern, anxiety, and worry." He therefore openly instructs public health officials how to effectively manipulate the public through biased media reports and various intimidation tactics. For example, the third step of his "recipe" suggests that "Medical experts and public health authorities publicly (e.g., via media) state concern and alarm (and predict dire outcomes) – and urge influenza vaccination." Step 5 further suggests "Continued reports (e.g., from health officials and media) that influenza is causing severe illness and/or affecting lots of people – helping foster the perception that many people are susceptible to a bad case of influenza." Nowak further advises, in steps 6 and 7, publicizing pictures of sick children and interviewing "families of those affected," in order to motivate the public, and to provide "references to, and discussions, of pandemic influenza." The "recipe" is expected to result in "Significant media interest and attention … in terms that motivate behavior (e.g. as 'very severe,' 'more severe than last or past years,' 'deadly')." What is especially concerning about this "recipe" is that, as the title of the presentation suggests, it was not designed as a localized solution to a specific disease, more serious than usual flu, which might have justified the use of intimidation in Novak's view. It was not even designed specifically for influenza vaccines. It was, as Novak himself articulated, a general formula, meaning that intimidation is a recommended tactic for any vaccine and at any time.

In the creation of the villain myth, another tactic used by health authorities is supplying the media with frequent updates on the progress of the epidemic, and on each death. Dew (1999) describes how during the 1985 measles epidemic in New Zealand, this frequent updating resulted in an intensive media report, focusing on the numbers of cases: "56 cases of measles one day, 125 cases two days later, 140 cases two days later, and so on" (Dew, 1999 p. 385). Similarly, during the 2009 H1N1 outbreak, the media were flooded with dramatic, sensational and frightening stories about people who contracted or died from the disease. The source of this media craze was the intensive reporting of the Israeli Health Ministry, through press releases disseminated among health journalists following each death (Alon, 2009). "Instead of calming the concerned public, the Ministry of Health published a press release each time someone died from swine flu," said Judy Siegel, the health correspondent of the *Jerusalem Post*. "I begged them not to do this. It is unnecessary."

This intense updating was accompanied by alarming predictions: "We are preparing for actual cases of death in Israel from swine flu in the coming days," stated Dr. Ran Blitzer, health adviser to the Health Ministry on influenza pandemic preparedness, in an interview to the media (Even et al., 2009).

Furthermore, while each death even suspected as related to the epidemic is reported meticulously, the circumstances that surround those deaths are not disclosed (Dew, 1999). For example, during the 1985 measles epidemic in New Zealand, two cases of death of children from measles were recorded and reported in the media. It turned out that one of these children had a non-Hodgkins lymphoma and was on chemotherapy, and contracted measles although having already been vaccinated. The other child had a mucolipidosis and developed a secondary bacterial infection (Butler, 1991). Similarly, during the 2009 H1N1 outbreak in Israel, some of the cases of death were attributed to the virus even before the cause of death was verified, and, although the patients suffered from severe comorbidities. For instance, in the first case of death reported, the Health Ministry rushed to update the media and stated that the patient, aged 35, died from swine flu, although at the time, the circumstances of his death were still unclear, given that the patient was a heavy smoker and was diagnosed with pneumonia. "We'll wait for the test results," said Dr. Itamar Grotto, head of the Public Health Services in the Israeli Ministry of Health, "but the data currently indicate that it was probably swine flu-related death" (Even et al., 2009). Similarly, the death of a 57-year-old man who suffered from severe comorbidities and was diagnosed with H1N1 was attributed to the virus (Talmor, 2009). In another case, the death of a 19-year-old man was attributed by the Health Ministry to H1N1, although he died two days after having fallen off a scaffolding from a height of 3 meters, suffering a severe head injury. Health Ministry officials insisted that since he was also diagnosed with H1N1and the reason for his fall was not clear, his death would be considered another case of H1N1-related death (Talmor, 2009).

### The knight in shining armor: the perfect vaccine

In the drug narrative, the disease is the villain and the drug is the hero – the brave knight riding a white horse, coming to the rescue of humankind. According to Lule (2001), the hero myth is the most widespread myth in the world. It is the manifestation of the core values and ideals in every society. Indeed, drugs make an ideal knight – 100% effective, with no side effects or risks. In the pharma's press releases, drugs are often presented as a warlord or general, who leads his army in a brave fight against the cruel enemy, defeats it and saves humanity (Shir-Raz, 2014).

To achieve this strategy, overly dramatic descriptions are again employed. For instance, stating that a certain drug "recruits the NK cells – the elite elimination unit of the immune system … to attack and eliminate invading cells." Alternatively, drugs are depicted as innovative weapons used by doctors, while in such cases, the doctors themselves are the heroes. For example, describing a certain drug as "a guided target missile which zeros on the tumor cells"; or "these are the most effective weapons in the hands of doctors."

This emotional appeal is, again, complemented by a cognitive approach. In this case this is carried out through the presentation of clinical studies in which the drug was examined, or, more precisely, of selective findings and data from those studies, chosen carefully to indicate efficiency and safety. Almost a quarter – 22.7% of the pharma's press releases present data from clinical studies. On the other hand, only 2.3% of the press releases mention side effects. Thus, similar to the depiction of the disease, the portrayal of drugs combines pathos and logos, which together create an illusion of a flawless solution.

The following examples demonstrate that this same strategy is adopted extensively by health organizations and officials to portray vaccines. In this case, the vaccine is the perfect solution to the problem – the outbreak (actual or potential). The vaccine is the brave knight who time and time again rescues humanity from a cruel and vicious enemy.

The first goal in constructing this perfect solution is to create an image of an incredibly effective vaccine. The HPV vaccine is a prominent example. The CDC website announces, "The HPV vaccine works extremely well" (CDC, 2015h), and that "The human papillomavirus (HPV) vaccines are safe, effective, and offer long-lasting protection against cancers caused by HPV" (CDC, 2015g). Other organizations are even more enthusiastic. On a website dedicated to this vaccine, Cancer Council Australia, a national non-government organization, which advises the Australian government and other bodies on practices and policies related to cancer, states: "The latest research shows the vaccine still offers close to 100% protection more than 5 years after it was received, and this protection shows no sign of weakening" (Cancer Council Australia, n.d.). But what does it mean to "work extremely well"? What exactly does the HPV vaccine offer close to 100% protection from? The impression created by such statements is that it is the ultimate solution for cervical cancer, and that it can even eliminate it. Yet, as Tomljenovic and Shaw (2013) argue, a closer examination of the data reveals that the long-term effects of the vaccine in preventing cancer have not been demonstrated. So far, studies have actually shown results that are more modest: efficacy in preventing infection by specific strains of HPV covered by the vaccine, and in protecting against pre-cancers caused by HPV strains covered by the vaccine genital warts (CDC, 2015h). As the National Women's Health Network (2015) acknowledges, "Additional research is needed to assess the vaccines' safety, long-term effects, and use in subgroups (like older women)." In addition, as the WHO and the CDC admit, none of the existing vaccines is able to clear existing infections or prevent their progression (CDC, 2015c; Cutts et al., 2007). Moreover, according to Tomljenovic and Shaw (2013), even if the vaccines prove effective against cervical cancer, there is no evidence that it would reduce cervical cancer rates beyond what pap screening has already achieved. Thus, they argue, the current worldwide HPV immunization practices are in fact based on what even the FDA acknowledges as assumptions regarding its the long-term benefits, rather than solid research data (Tomljenovic and Shaw, 2013).

The influenza vaccine receives similar treatment. Doshi (2013) argues that in addition to inflating the prevalence and severity of seasonal influenza, the CDC has been overstating the efficacy of influenza vaccines. As an example, Doshi cites a study presented in a CDC press briefing (CDC, 2013a), which indicated that the overall effectiveness of the influenza vaccines is 62%. Regarding this finding, CDC director Tom Frieden told reporters: "You can say 62 percent is certainly far less than we wish it would be. But it's a glass 62 percent full or a 62 percent reduction in the number of people who would be going to doctor's offices if they hadn't been vaccinated." Yet what the study did not reveal, since it did not present the statistics by age or health status, was the fact that 90% of the study's participants were younger than 65. Moreover, there was no significant benefit for older people. Since for certain groups of people, such as the older population, influenza infections are more severe compared with healthy young adults, this information is vital. Therefore, Doshi argues, there are good reasons to assume that this 62% reduction does not hold true for all subpopulations. He also criticizes the agency's use of observational studies that concluded that influenza vaccines can reduce the risk of the elderly of death from all causes by 27%–48%. Doshi (2013) claims:

> If true, these statistics indicate that influenza vaccines can save more lives than any other single licensed medicine on the planet. Perhaps there is a reason CDC does not shout this from the rooftop: it is too good to be true. Since at least 2005, non-CDC researchers have pointed out the seeming impossibility that influenza vaccines could be preventing 50% of all deaths from all causes when influenza is estimated to only cause around 5% of all wintertime deaths.

Indeed, accumulating evidence from large systematic reviews conducted by the Cochrane over the last decade indicates that those results *are* too good to be true. For instance, the most recent Cochrane meta-analysis of the effectiveness of vaccines for preventing influenza in healthy adults, which included 90 reports (Demicheli et al., 2014) concluded: "Influenza vaccines have a very modest effect in reducing influenza symptoms and working days lost in the general population, including pregnant women." Similar conclusions emerge from a previous analysis, which included 50 reports and focused on healthy adults as well (Jefferson et al., 2010b): "Influenza vaccines have a modest effect in reducing influenza symptoms and working days lost." Another review, which included 75 studies and focused on elderly people (Jefferson et al., 2010a) concluded that "The available evidence is of poor quality and provides no guidance regarding the safety, efficacy or effectiveness of influenza vaccines for people aged 65 years or older." Even more disturbing is the repeated warning the authors make in each of these reviews – that a large part of the trials included in them (i.e., a large part of the trials conducted in this field) are industry-funded, and some have no funding declaration. Furthermore, they warn, "Industry funded studies were published in more prestigious journals and cited more than other studies independently from methodological quality and size" (Jefferson et al., 2010b).

"We have few trials, and masses of very poor quality observational evidence," said Jefferson in an interview in *The Guardian* newspaper. "We have presented evidence of considerable reporting bias, which governments continue to ignore. The science is missing and so making an informed decision is very difficult" (Dillner, 2014).

The data provided by the CDC itself reveals that the vaccine effectiveness is far more modest than advertised by the agency, and although in some years it reaches 50%–60%, in others it is only 10%–23%. For instance, in 2004–2005 the benefit was only 10%; in 2005–2006, it was 21%; and in 2014–2015, it was 23% (CDC, 2016b). A major factor that can explain this modest effectiveness is the difficulty in matching the vaccine viruses to the circulating strains of influenza each year. The strains of influenza to be used in the vaccine each year are chosen several months before the flu season starts in order to give the manufacturers time to produce the vaccines. The match occasionally proves inaccurate. In 2014–2015, for example, the CDC admitted that "about half of the viruses" were different from the ones that were included in the vaccine, and as a result, the vaccine may not have offered as much protection as the experts had hoped (Sloane, 2014). However, Doshi argues, "even the ideal influenza vaccine, matched perfectly to circulating strains of wild influenza …, can only deal with a small part of the 'flu' problem" (2013, p. 3), since most reported flu cases are in fact not influenza, but rather other flu-like viruses.

In order to maintain the impression of a perfect solution, sometimes findings indicating inefficacy are withheld from the public, and even policy makers may be kept in the dark. A recent example is the discussion regarding Flumist, the nasal-spray influenza vaccine, held by the Advisory Committee on Infectious Diseases and Immunization in August 2015 in Israel. In February 2015, the U.S. Advisory Committee on Immunization Practices (ACIP – a panel of immunization experts that advises the CDC), voted to drop its 2014 guide-lines that indicated that the nasal-spray influenza vaccine (i.e., LAIV) should be preferred over injectable vaccines (i.e., IIV) for children aged 2–8. A CDC press release explained that the decision "was based on new data from more recent seasons which have not confirmed superior effectiveness of LAIV observed in earlier studies" (CDC, 2015b). These data came from three new studies (Caspard et al., 2016; Chung et al., 2016; Gaglani et al., 2016), one of which (Gaglani et al., 2016) showed no significant effectiveness of the nasal-spray influenza vaccine against influenza A (H1N1) among children in the 2013–2014 season, and the other two reported reduced effectiveness of nasal-spray influenza vaccine, compared with the injectable vaccines (Caspard et al., 2016; Chung et al., 2016). Although the press release does not mention these studies, it does clarify that "Data from the 2013–2014 season showed no measurable effectiveness for LAIV against influenza A (H1N1) among children." It also adds that interim data from the 2014–2015 season suggest that LAIV did not work better than IIV against the predominant H3N2 viruses circulating during that season, and that neither vaccine worked well in protecting against H3N2 viruses.

Similar to their American counterparts, the Israeli members of the Advisory Committee on Infectious Diseases and Immunization voted on August 2015 not to renew the recommendation for the nasal-spray vaccine over injectable vaccines for children for the 2015–2016 season. Yet, unlike the ACIP, the Israeli committee members deliberated if and how to explain this change to the public, finally deciding not to mention "the issue of the vaccine's effectiveness." While stressing their desire for transparent communication, the committee members thought it was best to keep the explanation "more simple and friendly," and focus on the "problem with the vaccine supply." Their main concern was that a statement focusing problems with the efficacy of the vaccine might "undermine" their recommendations to the Healthcare Basket, and ruin the chances of Flumist being included in 2016 Healthcare Basket (Israeli Ministry of Health, 2015f).

Omitting information that does not support the effectiveness of the vaccines reinforces the hero myth, creating a perfect solution capable of eliminating deadly diseases from the face of the planet. Dew (1999) argues that this imagery establishes goals that allow for no disagreement, and suggests that even if some people pay a price in terms of adverse effects – it is a price worth paying, since it is ultimately for the good of the whole community, and the entire world.

Yet, in an attempt to prevent damage to the status of vaccination programs, health authorities and officials make considerable efforts to suppress evidence of side effects and adverse events. A striking example is the following statement in an FDA guidance document:

> Although the continued availability of the vaccine may not be in immediate jeopardy, *any possible doubts, whether or not well founded, about the safety of the vaccine cannot be allowed to exist* in view of the need to assure that the vaccine will continue to be used to the maximum extent consistent with the nation's public health objectives.
>
> (FDA, 1984; emphasis added)

Pre-empting doubts about vaccine safety thus becomes a primary goal, and in order to achieve it, several of tactics are employed. A key tactic is aggregating all available data on the vaccine's side effects in the publications and guides for the public, while leaving out any information that might spark doubts or reservations. For example, in December 2011, the Israeli Advisory Committee on Infectious Diseases and Immunization convened to discuss the following question: to what extent should parents be informed about possible side effects caused by vaccines their children receive? (Israeli Ministry of Health, 2011). Some of the committee members thought that the first draft of the manual published earlier that year was "too detailed" and might therefore deter parents. They claimed the manual should only include common side effects, going as far as to dub severe but more rare side effects noted in the manufacturer's leaflet "unnecessary and misleading information": "It is our duty to protect the vaccines from this unnecessary and misleading information," determined one of the committee members. Moreover, it was further demanded that the side effects would be detailed "generically for every vaccine against a particular disease, rather than separately for each manufacturer," although the vaccine formulas made by different manufacturers tend to differ, causing different potential side effects. Ultimately, the committee decided to correct the guide, reducing the list of side effects written in the manufacturer's leaflet.

In the digital age, this aggregated information is presented on organization websites and social media feeds. The manner in which it is presented on those sites generates another tactic, which can be dubbed "redness in the injection site." This tactic involves an opening statement arguing that the vaccine is "extremely safe" (Collignon et al., 2010), followed by a list of minor side effects, such as redness, pain or swelling in the arm where the shot was given, while potential or even reported serious adverse events are omitted. The HPV vaccine is a striking example. Since it was first introduced, there have been persistent reports of post-HPV vaccine-linked autoimmunity, including Guillain-Barré Syndrome (Laino, 2009; Souayah et al., 2011) and autoimmune diseases, such as ovarian failure (Colafrancesco et al., 2013; Little and Ward, 2012, 2014), postural orthostatic tachycardia syndrome (POTS) with chronic fatigue (Tomljenovic et al., 2014), and other disabling syndromes of chronic neuropathic pain, fatigue, and autonomic dysfunction (Martínez-Lavín et al., 2015). Following the increasing number of reports, experts throughout the world have been calling to conduct more studies and improve post-marketing surveillance (Colafrancesco et al., 2013; Little and Ward, 2014). In 2013, Japan withdrew its recommendation for HPV vaccine, due to concerns from the public about adverse events, and in 2015, guidelines for the evaluation and management of symptoms that begin after HPV vaccine injection were issued to healthcare professionals (Chustecka, 2015). In Canada, researchers demanded immediate suspension of the HPV vaccination program until its safety was established (Dyer, 2015), and in India, researchers, doctors, public health and women rights organizations submitted a memorandum to the government, urging it to halt the inclusion of the HPV vaccine in the immunization program (The Hindu Business Line, 2015). Yet, despite all this, the CDC webpage on HPV vaccine safety mentions none of the potential adverse reactions suspected as linked to the vaccine, nor are the accumulating reports mentioned. Instead, the webpage states: "The HPV vaccine is very safe ... The most common side effects are usually mild" (CDC, 2015h). The side effects detailed include local pain, redness or swelling, fever, headache or feeling tired, nausea and muscle or joint pain. Two other side effects mentioned, which were reported throughout the world, are fainting and seizures – yet, they are described through a minimizing rhetoric. They were described as "Brief fainting spells and related symptoms (such as jerking movements)" that can occur after any medical procedure, including vaccination. In addition: "Sitting or lying down for about 15 minutes after a vaccination can help prevent fainting and injuries caused by falls."

Sometimes, the optimism stated by health authorities regarding the vaccine safety is even more pronounced. For instance, in October 2009, Anthony Fauci, the US NIAID Director, argued on a promotional YouTube video, that "the track record for serious adverse events is very good. It's very, very, very rare that you ever see anything that's associated with the vaccine that's a serious event" (Fauci, 2009). In Israel, during the national polio vaccination campaign in 2013, Roni Gamzu, then the Ministry of Health Director General, stated that the oral polio vaccine had "zero risk" (GLZ, 2013).

Yet, such optimism is exaggerated and misguided (Collignon et al., 2010), since no medicine or vaccine has zero risk or no side effects. A prime example of just how misguided an over optimistic characterization of vaccines can be is the AS03-adjuvanted H1N1 pandemic vaccine Pandemrix used during the 2009 H1N1 outbreak (EMEA, 2009).

Pandemrix (made by GlaxoSmithKline) was approved by the European Commission following the recommendations of the EMA in September 2009. According to the European Medicine Association (EMA), the approval was granted following six main studies, which included 180 healthy adults aged 18–60, 120 healthy elderly subjects, aged over 60, and 260 healthy children aged 6 months and 17 years (European Medicine Association, 2009). Soon afterwards, scientists, doctors and politicians throughout the world criticized the decision made by governments to purchase millions of doses of Pandemrix without waiting for proper safety testing. Their main concern was the adjuvants, which, they feared, could produce inoculation reactions, including long-term side effects. They voiced concerns, especially regarding their safety for children and pregnant women (Stafford, 2009). One of the experts was Michael Kochen, President of the German College of General Practitioners and Family Physicians, who told the *BMJ* that Germany's decision to purchase 50 million doses was "a large-scale experiment on the German population." Kochen expressed concerns especially regarding the adjuvant, arguing that the potential risks outweigh the benefits. He said he himself would not take the vaccine and advised his colleagues not to give it to patients (Stafford, 2009). After *Der Spiegel* news magazine revealed that the Federal Interior Ministry had bought 200,000 doses of Celvapan (made by Baxter), another H1N1 vaccine, which was adjuvant-free, to be used by top government officials, Kochen was joined by Frank Ulrich Montgomery, Vice-President of the German Medical Association, who called for adjuvant-free vaccinations for pregnant women and children (Stafford, 2009). Another German expert who criticized the H1N1 vaccination program was Wolf-Dieter Ludwig, Chairman of the German Medical Association's drug commission, who argued that neither Pandemrix nor Celvapan had been adequately tested (Stafford, 2009). In France, Dr. Marc Girard, a specialist in the side effects of drugs and a medical expert commissioned by French courts, told France 24 television that the "swine flu" vaccine was not just "badly developed" but "not developed," and could put many people in danger, especially young people, children and pregnant women (France 24, 2009). In Italy, the Deputy Health Minister, Ferruccio Fazio, and the Mayor of Rome, Gianni Alemanno, have decided against vaccination, and six out of every ten Italian family physicians refused to prescribe the A/H1N1 vaccine for their patients, claiming that the risks of the vaccine outweigh its benefits. Mario Nejrotti, the Director of torinomedica.com, said that a similar vaccine manufactured in the USA in 1976 had contributed to a considerable number of cases of Guillain-Barré syndrome (Press TV, 2009). In Poland, Health Minister Ewa Kopacz announced at a press conference that she refused to order H1N1 vaccines, explaining, "Their testing lasted a relatively short amount of time. It is not known whether [the vaccine] is safe for children and pregnant women" (Chowdhury, 2009). In Israel, Dr. Daizy Stern, a family and preventive medicine expert, wrote a letter to Professor Dan Engelhard, Head of the Israeli pandemic team, urging him to revoke the decision to use the two adjuvanted H1N1 vaccines – Pandemrix in children aged 3–10 and Focetria for adults. The letter, which was also published as an online petition to the Health Ministry, warned that the vaccine was not well studied, and that the adjuvant used in it might be toxic to the nervous system and cause severe autoimmune reactions, including death (Stern, 2009). Engelhard replied in a letter of his own, also published online, in various media outlets: "The [H1N1] influenza is dangerous and threatening – the vaccine is effective, safe and much recommended" (Engelhard, 2009). He rejected her arguments, claiming they are "scientifically baseless," and that the vaccine and the adjuvant were well studied and undoubtedly safe. In addition, the Health Ministry published a media release responding to Stern's letter, calling it "false information, unreliable and unprofessional" (Naim, 2009). Another expert, Dr. Efi Halperin, Head of the Infectious Diseases Unit in Bikur Holim Hospital in Jerusalem, criticized the Health Ministry's conduct during the H1N1 vaccination campaign, and he too, questioned the decision to use the adjuvant vaccines (Halperin, 2009). Halperin stressed that the adjuvanted H1N1 vaccines were not yet well studied, that they were not approved by the FDA (upon which the Israeli Health Ministry usually relies when approving drugs and vaccine), and that in Canada, 170,000 doses of the H1N1 vaccine Arepanrix, which is also an AS03-adjuvanted vaccine, were withdrawn after health officials announced there has been a higher-than-usual number of anaphylactic shock reactions (PreventDisease, 2009). The Ministry of Health responded to these arguments: "The claims indicate a lack of understanding and familiarity with the facts" (Halperin, 2009). Yet, a few months later, in 2010, Pandemrix was associated with a spike in cases of narcolepsy among adolescents in Sweden and in Finland. Subsequent investigations by the European Medicines Agency, the Swedish Medical Products Agency and a cohort study in Finland reported a 13-fold increased risk of narcolepsy after vaccination in children and young people aged 4–19, most of whom had onset within three months after vaccination and almost all within six months (Nohynek et al., 2012). The association of Pandemrix vaccination and narcolepsy in children and adolescents had also been reported in Sweden, Norway, Ireland, France, and the UK (ANSM, 2012; Heier et al., 2013; Miller et al., 2013; National Narcolepsy Study Steering Committee, 2012). In adults, the Pandemrix vaccination was associated with narcolepsy in Sweden, Finland and France (ANSM, 2012; Persson et al., 2014). The Finnish National Institute for Health and Welfare, as well as non-governmental researchers, confirmed the vaccine's role in these serious adverse events (European Medicines Agency, 2011; Medical Products Agency, 2010, 2011; Miller et al., 2013; Vaarala et al., 2014).

Thus, health authorities aggregate all available information on each of the side effects of the vaccines. The aggregated data is presented to the public as "facts," coupled with a decisive statement arguing that the vaccine is "very safe" and involves merely minor side effects, or in some cases, using even more positive proclamations, such as "zero side effects." Consequently, these combined tactics generate information that is then conveyed by policy-makers and experts as the "scientific truth." The public, and even the medical community, may find it difficult to judge this "truth," making doubts unlikely. In cases where doubts or questions nevertheless arise, they are firmly opposed, often while attacking the person raising them, whether it is a concerned parent, a journalist or even an expert.

### *The epidemic narrative or "epidemic mongering"*

Foucault wrote that the representation of diseases is the product of a social setting and of the relationships between power and knowledge (Foucault, 1972, 1977). These relationships, according to Foucault (1980), allow those in power to impose their own ideology, using scientific discourse, which has a special status in technologically-advanced countries, to turn this ideology into "truth." The numerous examples presented in this chapter demonstrate how, in order to impose this "scientific truth" regarding outbreaks and vaccines and disseminate it effectively among the public and the medical community, health authorities do not make do with scientific discourse. They resort to use of both "science" – the cognitive appeal, or "logos," suggested by Aristotle, as well as the emotional appeal – "pathos." Employing these two approaches, health authorities present the "problem" and its "solution" through two of the fundamental myths in every human society – the "villain" and the "hero." Together, these two myths create "the epidemic narrative," i.e., the epidemic is extremely dangerous, but not to worry, the vaccine will save you. Instead of a means for promoting the important goal of preventing deadly infectious diseases, immunization status has become the Holy Grail – the goal itself, which must be promoted by means of every possible communication strategy.

As this chapter demonstrates, the strategies and tactics used are surprisingly similar to those used by the pharmaceutical industries in order to promote their products. As another document summarizing a meeting of the Israeli Advisory Committee on Infectious Diseases and Immunization states, the most efficient way authorities see fit is "to improve the immunization status using medical propagandizing" (Israeli Ministry of Health, 2008).

Nevertheless, perhaps it is not so surprising that authorities adopt the pharma's strategies, given many years of working together with the industry. There is no doubt that the ultimate goal of preventing fatal infectious diseases is important, and that to promote this goal, it is necessary to work together. Nevertheless, adopting the pharma's strategies might lead to what Goldacre calls "a regulatory capture" – "the process whereby a state regulator ends up promoting the interests of the industry it is supposed to monitor, at the expense of the public interest" (Goldacre, 2013, p. 123). The CDC's "recipe" for generating demand for vaccination is a glaring example. In an interview on National Public Radio (NPR), Nowak explained that the reason the agency decided to adopt this strategy was that the demand for vaccines during the 2003 season was low. "At that point, the manufacturers were telling us that they weren't receiving a lot of orders for vaccine for use in November or even December [of 2003] … It really did look like we needed to do something to encourage people to get a flu shot" (Doshi, 2005).

Characterizing an infectious disease as a dangerous threat, while promoting the vaccine as a risk-free solution, creates the "epidemic narrative." These same tactics have been described by Lynn Payer as "disease mongering" (Payer, 1992). Payer's definition related primarily to the pharmaceutical companies, which sell sickness in order to expand the market for their products. Unfortunately, too many examples demonstrate that the strategies used by health authorities to raise public awareness of various infectious diseases and promote immunization are worthy of this definition as much as the pharma's marketing strategies. The only differences are that in this case, as Doshi (2013) concludes, the salesmen are public health officials, and the diseases sold are epidemics. Thus, promoting vaccination by sowing fear becomes "epidemic mongering."

## Part 4 From no proven causal relationship to no relationship

Statistics have been the dominant scientific method for shaping public health policies since World War II (CDC, 2012a), and have been used in epidemiology since John Graunt's landmark analysis of mortality data published in 1662

(Bernstein, 1998). The purpose of using statistics is to determine causal relationships, or alternatively, to prove lack of causal relationship, based on the idea that the assessment bears statistic strength and is therefore statistically significant.

In the age of "Big Data" there is a vast amount of information, and consequently, a far greater number of factors. Thus, the critical question that arises is: is there a "statistically significant" way to prove causal factors? Simply put, in a complex world full of uncertainty, is it really possible to prove causality through the lens of *P* value? (Garcia-Berthou and Alcaraz, 2004; Jeng, 2006). This question must be examined by researchers and scientists, as well as health policy-makers who formulate opinion papers and guidelines according to epidemiological and clinical studies. Can the statistical methods used today provide the answers we need? What other alternatives are there? These questions need to be examined in the framework of the future of the science of public health. With regard to risk communication, this is the decisive question. Here we ask: How do authorities communicate the topic of causality? How does this type of communication affect the public's comprehension and behavior?

Many studies focus on the issue of epidemiology. In particular, there is increasing criticism of how researchers reach conclusions by examining the strength of a causal relationship. As Goodman has argued:

> The standard statistical approach has created this situation by promoting the illusion that conclusions can be produced with certain "error rates," without consideration of information from outside the experiment. This statistical approach, the key components of which are *P* values and hypothesis tests, is widely perceived as a mathematically coherent approach to inference.
>
> (1999, p. 995)

Furthermore, the controversy surrounding the statistical test of *P* values has intensified to the point that in 2015, the editors of *Basic and Applied Social Psychology* (BASP) announced that the journal would no longer publish articles containing *P* values because the statistics were too often used to support lower-quality research (Trafimow and Marks, 2015). In an interview in the journal, *Nature*, Trafimow said that he would be happy if the test disappeared from all published research: "If scientists are depending on a process that's blatantly invalid, we should get rid of it" (Woolston, 2015).

Sterne and Smith (2001) have concluded that medical research must advance forward from the idea that results are significant or nonsignificant to the interpretation of findings in the context of the type of study and other available evidence, and suggest new approaches for reporting and interpretation.

Many studies have shown that epidemiological and clinical studies of medicines that indicated statistical significance have ultimately been found to be misleading. A striking example is the decision taken by governments throughout the world to stock up on anti-viral drugs in the event of an epidemic. This decision was influenced by the claims that anti-viral drugs are beneficial for lowering the risk of complications from influenza. The USA has spent more than $1.3 billion on building up a strategic reserve of these drugs (GAO, 2011), and the British government has paid out almost £424 million to stock up on 40 million doses (House of Commons Committee of Public Accounts, 2014).

Regarding the anti-flu drugs, Tamiflu and Relenza (both of which constitute the same antiviral medication), it has been shown that both reduce flu symptoms only by about half a day compared to a placebo (Jefferson et al., 2014). Taking Tamiflu or Relenza leads to a reduction in symptoms from 6.3 to 7 days in adults; and in children no changes were found. Moreover, there has been no evidence to support the claims that these drugs reduce the amount of hospitalizations or chances of severe complications resulting from the flu, nor do they prevent contracting the flu in the first place. However, it has been shown that taking these drugs increases one's chances of suffering from side effects such as nausea and vomiting. In studies in which the drugs were given to prevent the flu, it has been shown that they increased side effects, such as headaches, psychiatric episodes and liver complications. Similarly, evidence has shown that in some people, the drug prevents the body from creating natural antibodies that fight infection. This case exemplifies the problematic nature of reliance on epidemiological studies as the sole source for policy making.

For many years, epidemiology has been seen as the Holy Grail of science – the discipline upon which scientific studies rely, leading to far-reaching conclusions. As John P. Ioannidis (2005) has articulated:

> There is increasing concern that most current published research findings are false. The probability that a research claim is true may depend on study power and bias, the number of other studies on the same question, and, importantly, the ratio of true to no relationships among the relationships probed in each scientific field.

This claim has been echoed by various studies (Collaborative Group on Hormonal Factors in Breast Cancer, 2002). The *British Medical Journal* devoted an editorial to the problem of evidence-gathering in the field of epidemiology, arguing that recent randomized control trials have supported the widespread perception that epidemiological studies generate conflicting and often meaningless findings (Smith and Ebrahim, 2002). The literature on the limits of epidemiological research has considered the phenomenon of "false positive" findings that has been identified in the research conducted by many professionals (epidemiologists, doctors, statisticians). This phenomenon can be explained by the presence of many causal relationships. The magnitude of findings allows professionals to manipulate the numbers in order to find an association that seems significant (The Alpha-Tocopherol Beta Carotene Cancer Prevention Study Group, 1994). When a large number of relationships appear in a dataset where only a few real associations exist, a *P* value of 0.05 is compatible with the large majority of findings still being false positives. Traditionally, a study is said to be "statistically significant" if the odds are only 1 in 20 that the result could be pure chance. Yet in a field where there are many potential hypotheses to sift through – such as whether a particular gene influences a particular disease – it is easy to reach false conclusions using this method. If you test 20 false hypotheses, one of them is likely to show up as true, on average (Ioannidis, 2005). In addition, Simmons, Nelson, and Simonsohn (2011) raise other possible causes of false positive findings. One such factor is the tendency of prestigious journals not to publish null findings, giving researchers little incentive to submit them.

Another reason for false positive findings is that drug companies themselves will not submit research findings to journals if those findings do not support the efficacy of the drug (Bero et al., 2007; Bourgeois et al., 2010; Turner et al., 2008; Yaphe et al., 2001). This practice elicits a "closed circle" and leads to deception within the field of epidemiology, using significant statistical associations and evidence for causality. Criticism has led to attempts to correct this bias, such as steps taken by an international committee of journal editors (ICMJE), which demanded that clinical trials be registered in a database of clinical trials as a condition for being published in a medical journal. They went so far as to announce that clinical trials not registered in the database would not be accepted for publication (Laine et al., 2007). These steps led the FDA to amend the law in 2007, such that protocol abstracts of clinical trials had to be registered through a site (www.clinicaltrials.gov) within a year of completion. However, a 2012 study published in the *British Medical Journal* revealed that the amendment did not solve the problem, since only 22% of clinical trials actually reported results within a year (Prayle et al., 2012). The consequences of not reporting all clinical trials is epitomized in the findings of the *Cochrane Review*, which found that 60% of the information found in studies on Tamiflu was never actually published (Godlee, 2012). Only after a protracted struggle that lasted more than four years did the editor of the *BMJ*, Dr. Fiona Godlee, receive all the available information from the findings of studies on Tamiflu (The Cochrane Collaboration, 2014).

A vast literature has examined the issue of deception and bias in epidemiological findings, revealing how studies indicate allegedly positive effects of a certain drug and highlight an association between the drug and its positive effects. While this phenomenon has been described in many methodological studies, the professional literature has paid less attention to the phenomenon of negative side effects that occur after taking a particular drug or after exposure to a particular toxin. Studies on negative side effects of vaccines or drugs, or on the consequences of exposure to toxins, tend to argue that causal association cannot be definitively proven. Similarly, epidemiological researchers tend to express reservations or criticism regarding alternatives to illness prevention, other than the drugs offered by the pharmaceutical industry proper. We would like to suggest that some researchers who try to show positive causal relationships in their studies express reservations when it comes to showing a causal relationship regarding negative side effects, or a causal relationship regarding the efficacy of products that do not promote the pharmaceutical industry.

In light of the complexity of the issue of causality, researchers have attempted to allocate specific criteria for relative risk. There are many reasons for this complexity. Here we would like to address one of the main reasons, namely, the difficulty in applying statistical methodology, which refers to the averages drawn from groups of people, to a single biological individual. Rothman and Greenland have emphasized the need to pinpoint many risk factors that may cause an individual to become ill, including genetic, environmental, and behavioral factors. According to them,

> Tobacco smoking is a cause of lung cancer, but by itself it is not a sufficient cause ... smoking even defined explicitly, will not cause cancer in everyone ... it is apparent from epidemiological data that some people can engage in chain smoking for many decades without developing cancer.
>
> (Rothman and Greenland, 2002)

For this reason, McElduff, Attia, Ewald, Cockburn, and Heller (2002) conclude that the uncertainty inherent in the individual biological model leads to a difficulty in pinpointing causality. "Causal pathway: In the absence of details biological model we assume that each risk factor is individually sufficient, but not necessary for causation of the outcome." Susser (1977) has pointed out that statistical association is a quantitative criterion and is measurable, but its significance and use depend on the researcher's own reasoning: "While strength of association is a quantitative criterion, its application requires judgment."

Epidemiology cannot indicate "definite causes" of diseases. The best that epidemiology can provide is a probability statement (Golan and Linn, 2015). From this perspective, we can argue that in clinical trials that test drugs on humans, there are biological factors that cause drugs to affect different people in different ways, even if we take into consideration confounders and standardizations. It is not possible to definitively isolate these effects. Furthermore, more than one set of components may be sufficient for the same effect. Although we are referring to the complexity of the same mechanism, when we are talking about efficacy of drugs or vaccines, there is a tendency in the scientific literature to indicate a positive association. When it comes to what we have called "damages," there are reservations with regard to proving a positive causal relationship. This is despite the fact that with regard to damages (side effects), epidemiological research can estimate only the lower degree of risk that exists between a risk factor and an illness. There is a significant likelihood that the greatest damage would be caused by the scientific estimate in and of itself. In other words, science indicates an underestimation of the risk.

This type of misclassification, as long as it occurs randomly, along with any sort of random error, serves to lower the risk estimate. Therefore, any epidemiological qualitative estimate regarding a positive association cannot negate a positive association. Moreover, it is sometimes impossible to find a specific risk factor. At the same time, the absence of a specific factor does not negate causality. As Rothman has emphasized, "The existence of one effect of an exposure dose not detract from the possibility that another effect exists" (Rothman and Greenland, 2005). Statistical significance is therefore a standard for estimating the percentage of error in scientific reasoning according to an arbitrary determination of a false positive rate that we can accept or reject, but this does not indicate that the factor is definitely the cause – it only reflects probability. This leads to the claim that statistical significance cannot be the only criterion in determining biological causality. If someone is exposed to a particular drug known for causing side effects or damages, this leads to the "precautionary principle" of the WHO (Martuzzi and Ticknet, 2004). Shai Lin, "Proof of causal relationship regarding a patient exposed to carcinogen, versus proof of excess morbidity in a group that was exposed to a material of unknown content" Medicine and Law 41 (December 2009). This is applied only partially, especially with regard to environmental issues in public health, but is not applied in other branches of public health. Despite the limitations inherent in applying statistical methods, health authorities nevertheless continue to use them in an absolute way, ignoring other sources, including qualitative and quantitative methodologies in order to overcome real uncertainty and gaps in scientific knowledge.

We would like to point out several of the organizations' communication strategies tactics for communicating issues regarding side effects or discussing factors that cause diseases.

### Doubt is their product

The primary strategy is what David Michaels has called "manufacturing uncertainty." In his book, *Doubt Is Their Product* (2008), Michaels describes how industries and scientists recruited by them "manufactured uncertainty by questioning every study, dissecting every method, and disputing every conclusion." Using hundreds of documents, Michaels demonstrates how the strategy of "manufacturing uncertainty," through tactics developed by the tobacco industries, helps corporations prevent independent studies from indicating side effects or damages connected to their product. Unfortunately, casting doubt is also the central communication strategy used by health organizations, and the one from which all other strategies draw. The strategy revolves around the argument that there are biological, genetic, and environmental factors that affect a person's morbidity (Shrader-Frechette, 1996). Thus, it is not possible to single out one factor as a cause for a side effect of a drug or vaccine. As Michaels puts it:

> Some of these studies sound reasonably plausible, whereas some are sound indicators, but all of them were motivated by the same principle:

Find other causes for disease, find smokers who do not have disease, find new associations of whatever sort ... Also and always contest the methods that epidemiologists used. Argue that "expectation-led" interviewers bias results.

(2008, p. 9)

Researchers on epidemiology have searched for years for what is known as "confounders." This has led scientific research to criticize studies that do not consider the whole picture. A classic example is the studies sponsored by tobacco companies that have shown that there are factors other than smoking that cause lung cancer (Proctor, 2012; TIRC, 1964). Although this is a well-known strategy used by the industry, it nevertheless leads to undeniable conflicts of interest, which are sometimes difficult to overcome. This strategy has influenced, prevented and deferred regulation and policy making. The industry's goal was to foment inherent uncertainty in epidemiological studies, in order to forestall regulatory action. As Michaels contends: "Some of the scientific research that the industry conducts or funds is manipulated to *mask* rather than *find* exposure – disease relationships – that is, to protect corporations, not their workers" (2008, p. 70).

There are many examples of the industry's successes in using epidemiological tools through "litigation protection" in the form of endless debates that forestall regulatory action (Michaels, 2008, pp. 75–80, 176–191). They use scientific tools to carry this out, encouraging colleagues to use epidemiological tools to prevent the organizations from declaring damages or enforcing regulation. This strategy, which stems from the industry itself, pervades and influences health organizations in diverse ways. In what follows, we would like to discuss the most prevalent.

### Side-effects as "misconceptions"

One of the main strategies found on several health organizations' websites, is framing vaccine side effects as "misconceptions" or as "myths." In doing so, the strategic choice is to present all of the vaccines as one monolithic group, despite the diversity of vaccines and side effects.

For example, the following document presented on the WHO website, entitled "Six common misconceptions about immunization," explains:

Vaccines are actually very safe, despite implications to the contrary in many anti-vaccine publications. Most vaccine adverse events are minor and temporary, such as a sore arm or mild fever. These can often be controlled by taking paracetamol after vaccination. More serious adverse events occur rarely (on the order of one per thousands to one per millions of doses), and some are so rare that risk cannot be accurately assessed. As for vaccines causing death, again so few deaths can plausibly be attributed to vaccines, that it is hard to assess the risk statistically. Each death reported to ministries of health is generally thoroughly examined to assess whether it is really related to administration of vaccine, and if so, what exactly is the cause. When, after careful investigation, an event is felt to be a genuine vaccine-related event, it is most frequently found to be a programmatic error, not related to vaccine manufacture.

(WHO, 2016a)

Another example, presented on the California Department of Public Health website, opens with the following statement: "California Department of Public Health Director Dr. Mark Horton addresses misconceptions about vaccines." This document lists "myths" vs. "facts":

MYTH #1: Vaccines aren't safe.
FACT: Vaccines are held to the highest standard of safety. Extensive testing is required by law before a vaccine can be licensed. Once in use, vaccines are continually monitored for safety and effectiveness. The United States currently has the safest, most effective vaccine supply in history.

(Horton, 2010)

### *A logical leap*

Another primary tactic is what we dub "a logical leap." It illustrates how "no relationship has been proven" becomes "there is no causal relationship." This is often the case when there is a medicine, a procedure or a vaccine, the safety of which is under debate in the scientific literature. A prominent example is the HPV vaccine. Some medical associations choose not to emphasize the element of uncertainty, instead affirming the research that has *not proven* a causal relationship between the vaccine and particular side effects, and framing this finding as "no relationship." For example, Laino (2009), and Souayah et al. (2011) found an increased risk for Guillain-Barré syndrome (GBS) after receiving the HPV vaccine. Nevertheless, the American Academy of Neurology chose to present a different study, which did not find an increase in Guillain-Barré syndrome after the HPV vaccination, and framed the findings as follows: "There is no causal relationship." They stated that, "The HPV vaccine does not increase the risk of developing Guillain-Barré syndrome, according to a study released today" (AAN, 2009; Jeffrey, 2009). Furthermore, this statement ignores another important finding reported in the same study – that when the date of vaccination is known, three-quarters of the probable cases of GBS in the database were reported within six weeks of the vaccination. This purposeful disregard is particularly striking in light of the fact that the study's authors themselves concluded that this finding "warrants continuous and careful analysis of GBS after vaccination with Gardasil" (AAN, 2009).

Moreover, several cases of onset or exacerbation of autoimmune diseases, such as ovarian failure (Colafrancesco et al., 2013) following the vaccine, have been reported in the literature and pharmacovigilance databases, triggering concerns about its safety. Following those cases, Pellegrino et al. (2014) analyzed and reviewed all case reports and studies dealing with either the onset of an autoimmune disease in vaccinated subjects or the safety in patients with autoimmune diseases, and concluded that solid evidence of causal relationship was provided in several cases in the studies they examined. Nevertheless, an information leaflet for parents issued jointly by the CDC, the American Academy of Family Physicians, and the American Academy of Pediatrics (CDC, 2016a) disregards these studies and instead, chooses to cite two other studies that did not find a link between autoimmune disorders and the HPV vaccines (Gardasil) (Chao et al., 2012; Grimaldi-Bensouda et al., 2014; Scheller et al., 2015). Furthermore, instead of stating that these studies did not *find* a causal relationship, the CDC's leaflet states: "Several studies have shown that there is no relationship between Gardasil and autoimmune disorders" (CDC, 2016a, p. 2).

### Many causes

Another tactic is the use of vague, noncommittal language when communicating risk. The communication on the subject of the HPV vaccine exemplifies this tactic. One of the side effects noted after giving this vaccination was fainting. In their communication on this subject, health organizations did not negate the possibility of a causal relationship between the vaccine and fainting. However, they open with a sentence that states that fainting can be caused by many factors, including vaccination, thereby indicating a possible causal relationship in vague, noncommittal terms. The WHO website issued the following statement:

> *Do people faint after getting HPV vaccines? People faint for many reasons.* Some preteens and teen may faint after any medical procedure, including receiving vaccines. It is possible for falls and injuries to occur after fainting. Sitting or lying down for about 15 minutes after a vaccination can help prevent fainting and related injuries.

(WHO, 2013b)

### Shifting the focus to other causes

A fourth strategy is shifting the focus to another possible cause of the side effect and, in so doing, denying a causal relationship between the vaccine and the side effect under debate. For instance, a media article reporting on a conference held by the European Society of Gynecology in 2008 presented "8 Myths about the Vaccine for Cervical Cancer." It cited several experts who spoke at the conference, explaining that, "Contrary to what you might have thought, cervical cancer vaccine is efficacious in Israel as well, is not dangerous, offers protection for a relatively long period, and is recommended by the European Society of Gynecology."

One of the experts cited in the article was Dr. Efraim Siegler, the head of the Cervix Clinic at the Carmel Medical Center and the President of the Israeli Society of Colposcopy and Cervical Pathology. He was quoted as saying:

> There were reports of someone who took contraceptive pills who received the vaccine, and she developed an aneurism. However, there is no indication that this was a result of the vaccine, given that contraceptive pills increase the risk of aneurism. In Australia, it was reported that ten girls fainted after receiving the vaccine, but it turned out that the reason was prolonged exposure to the sun while standing on line to receive the vaccine in the schoolyard.

Shifting the focus to another possible cause of the side effect – in this case, prolonged exposure to the sun, diverts attention from the vaccine to another possible cause, and thus helps eliminate any possible causal relationship between the vaccine and the side effect under discussion.

### Consequences of the communication of causal discourse on the public

Professionals, including scientists, regulators and risk managers, do not always agree with the public on the acceptable magnitude of a particular risk. Industry and government standards deem a certain level of risk to be safe (Bennett et al., 2010, pp. 49–50), that is, unlikely to cause harm to most people who lead a particular lifestyle. In contrast, the public demands minimum or no risk.

This mental gap between the organizations and the public might lead to situations in which the organizations' calls to vaccinate for public well-being or for altruistic reasons could fall on deaf ears. Alternatively, in order to mitigate the mental gap between the authorities and the public, organizations may sometimes use non-scientific language and declare a risk to be negligible or non-existent.

In addition, as noted above, organizations tend to adopt positivistic studies regarding drugs, maintaining skepticism regarding side effects. This tendency leads to two consequences. The first is that in doing so, the organizations legitimize the promotion and marketing of vaccines, without reliably communicating the risks, even when studies indicate that certain risks do exist. The second consequence results from the fact that the public is often ill-equipped to distinguish between reliable studies and industry-funded studies that aim to promote a commercial message. As a result, the public is often confused and helpless in the face of contradictory information. Moreover, the organizations sometimes act as an extension of the industry, rather than telling the public that no "causal relationship has been found" does not necessarily imply that there is "no relationship," in order to forestall regulation or prevent critical public discourse about the side effect indicated in studies.

The authorities' role is not to serve as an extension of the industry. However, their role is not to facilitate epidemiologists' and doctors' criticism of each other's studies using statistics shaped by the investigators' subjective assumptions and beliefs. We believe that, the organizations' task is to facilitate integration of all existing studies, in a way conducive to communicating findings with full transparency.

## References

AAN. (2009). Researchers: Guillain-Barré syndrome after HPV vaccine needs monitoring. Press release, February 13. Minneapolis, MN: American Academy of Neurology.

Adams, J. (1995). *Risk*. London: UCL Press.

Alaszewski, A. (2005). Risk communication: Identifying the importance of social context. *Health, Risk and Society*, 7(2), 101–105.

Alhakami, A. S., and Slovic, P. (1994). A psychological study of the inverse relationship between perceived risk and perceived benefit. *Risk Analysis*, 14(6), 1085–1096.

Alon, G. (2009). To calm or to alert? *Z'man Harefuah*, December 2009–January 2010.

ANSM. (2012). Pandemic influenza vaccine (H1N1) and narcolepsy: Results from the European study and the French case-control study – Information Point. September 20. Available at: http://ansm.sante.fr/S-informer/Points-d-information-Points-d-informa tion/Vaccins-pandemiques-grippe-A-H1N1-et-narcolepsie-Resultats-de-l-etude-europ eenne-et-de-l-etude-cas-temoins-francaise-Point-d-information (accessed May 6, 2016).

Arnst, C. (2006). Hey, you don't look so good. As diagnoses of once-rare illnesses soar, doctors say drugmakers are disease-mongering to boost sales. *Bloomberg Business*. May 8.

Aronson, S. S., and Shope, T. R. (2008). Outbreaks, epidemics, and other infectious disease emergencies. In S. S. Aronson and T. R. Shope (Eds.), *Managing Infectious Diseases in Child Care and Schools: A Quick Reference Guide*, 2nd Edition (pp. 169–171). Elk Grove Village, IL: American Academy of Pediatrics.

Associated Press. (2013). Top 10 newspapers by circulation: Wall Street Journal leads weekday circulation . *Huffington Post*, April 30. Available at: www.gutenberg.us/a rticles/list_of_newspapers_in_the_united_states_by_circulation

Baliga, S., and Sjöström, T. (2008). Strategic ambiguity and arms proliferation. *Journal of Political Economy*, 116(6), 1023–1057.

Bennett, P., Calman, K., Curtis, S., and Fischbacher-Smith, D. (2010). *Risk Communication and Public Health*, 2nd edition. Oxford: Oxford University Press.

Bernstein, P. L. (1998). *Against the Gods: The Remarkable Story of Risk*. New York: John Wiley & Sons, Inc.

Bero, L., Oostvogel, F., Bacchetti, P., and Lee, K. (2007). Factors associated with findings of published trials of drug-drug comparisons: Why some statins appear more efficacious than others. *PLoS Med*, 4(6), e184.

Bourgeois, F. T., Murthy, S., and Mandl, K. D. (2010). Outcome reporting among drug trials registered in ClinicalTrials.gov. *Annals of Internal Medicine*, 153(3), 158–166.

Bultmann, R. (1984). *New Testament Mythology and Other Basic Writings*. Minneapolis, MN: Fortress Press.

Butler, H. (1991). Measles: Who are you going to believe? *Options*, pp. 13–15. Available at: www.beyondconformity.co.nz/_literature_26498/Bio_HO_1991

Cancer Council Australia. (n.d.) HPV vaccine: How effective is the vaccine? Available at: www.hpvvaccine.org.au/the-hpv-vaccine/how-effective-is-the-vaccine.aspx (accessed May 2, 2016).

Caspard, H., Gaglani, M., Clipper, L., Belongia, E. A., McLean, H. Q., Griffin, M. R. et al. (2016). Effectiveness of live attenuated influenza vaccine and inactivated influenza vaccine in children 2–17 years of age in 2013–2014 in the United States. *Vaccine*, 34(1), 77–82.

CDC. (2012a). Principles of epidemiology in public health practice, third edition: An introduction to applied epidemiology and biostatistics. Lesson 1: Introduction to Epidemiology. Section 2: Historical evolution of epidemiology. Available at: www. cdc.gov/ophss/csels/dsepd/ss1978/lesson1/section2.html (accessed May 18, 2016).

CDC. (2012b). Principles of epidemiology in public health practice, third edition: An introduction to applied epidemiology and biostatistics. Lesson 6: Investigating an outbreak, Section 2: Steps of an outbreak investigation. Available at: www.cdc.gov/ ophss/csels/dsepd/ss1978/lesson6/section2.html (accessed February 18, 2016).

CDC. (2013a). Press briefing transcript: CDC update: Flu season and vaccine effectiveness. January 11, 2013. Available at: www.cdc.gov/media/releases/2013/t0111_ flu_season.html (accessed May 2, 2016).

CDC. (2013b). Press briefing transcript. Measles press conference: 50th anniversary of measles vaccine. December 5, 2013. Available at: www.cdc.gov/media/releases/2013/ t1205-measles-threat.html (accessed April, 30, 2016).

CDC. (2015a). Transcript for CDC Telebriefing: Measles in the United States, 2015. January 29, 2015. Available at: www.cdc.gov/media/releases/2015/t0129-measles-i n-us.html (accessed February 12, 2015).

CDC. (2015b). Advisory Committee on Immunization Practices (ACIP) reaffirms recommendation for annual influenza vaccination. February 26, 2015. Available at: www.cdc.gov/media/releases/2015/s0226-acip.html (accessed May 6, 2016).

CDC. (2015c). Epidemiology and prevention of vaccine-preventable diseases: Human papillomavirus. Available at: www.cdc.gov/vaccines/pubs/pinkbook/hpv.html (accessed May 2, 2016).

CDC. (2015d). Misconceptions about seasonal flu and flu vaccines: Questions and answers. Available at: www.cdc.gov/flu/about/qa/misconceptions.htm (accessed April 28, 2016).

CDC. (2015e). Flu vaccination coverage, United States, 2014–2015 influenza season. Available at: www.cdc.gov/flu/pdf/fluvaxview/nfid-coverage-2014-15-final.pdf (accessed April 29, 2016).

CDC. (2015f). Human papillomavirus (HPV). Available at: www.cdc.gov/hpv/ (accessed May 1, 2016).

CDC. (2015g). Human papillomavirus (HPV): HPV vaccine safety. Available at: www. cdc.gov/hpv/

CDC. (2015h). Human papillomavirus (HPV): Questions and answers. Available at: www.cdc.gov/hpv/parents/questions-answers.html (accessed May 2, 2016).

CDC. (2016a). Information for parents: HPV vaccine is safe – (Gardasil). Available at: www.cdc.gov/vaccinesafety/pdf/data-summary-hpv-gardasil-vaccine-is-safe.pdf (accessed May 6, 2016).

CDC. (2016b). Seasonal influenza vaccine effectiveness, 2005–2016. Available at: www. cdc.gov/flu/professionals/vaccination/effectiveness-studies.html (accessed May 6, 2016).

CDC and NFID. (2015). #FightFlu with a flu vaccine. Available at: www.thunderclap. it/projects/30520-fightflu-with-a-flu-vaccine (accessed May 1, 2016).

Chao, C., Klein, N. P., Velicer, C. M., et al. (2012). Surveillance of autoimmune conditions following routine use of quadrivalent human papillomavirus vaccine. *Journal of Internal Medicine*, 271(2), 193–203.

Chowdhury, S. (2009). Polish Health Minister Ewa Kopacz on the swine flu vaccine. YouTube, November 7. Available at: www.youtube.com/watch?v=xbtA6Lz-rA0 (accessed May 6, 2015).

Christley, R. M., Mort, M., Wynne, B., et al. (2013). "Wrong, but useful": negotiating uncertainty in infectious disease modelling. *PLoS One*, 8(10), e76277.

Chung, J. R., Flannery, B., Thompson, M. G., et al. (2016). Seasonal effectiveness of live attenuated and inactivated influenza vaccine. *Pediatrics*, 137(2).

Chustecka, Z. (2015). Japan scheme for managing symptoms after HPV vaccine. Available at: www.medscape.com/viewarticle/850436 (accessed May 6, 2016).

Clinton, H. (2015). The science is clear: The earth is round, the sky is blue, and #vaccineswork. Let's protect all our kids. Available at: #GrandmothersKnowBest.

Colafrancesco, S., Perricone, C., Tomljenovic, L., and Shoenfeld, Y. (2013). Human Papilloma Virus vaccine and primary ovarian failure: Another facet of the autoimmune/inflammatory syndrome induced by adjuvants. *American Journal of Reproductive Immunology*, 70(4), 309–316.

Collaborative Group on Hormonal Factors in Breast Cancer. (2002). Alcohol, tobacco and breast cancer – collaborative reanalysis of individual data from 53 epidemiological studies, including 58 515 women with breast cancer and 95 067 women without the disease. *British Journal of Cancer*, 87(11), 1234–1245.

Collignon, P., Doshi, P., and Jefferson, T. (2010). Adverse events following influenza vaccination in Australia–should we be surprised? Rapid response to Australia suspends seasonal flu vaccination of young children. *BMJ*, 340, c2419.

Connell, E., and Hunt, A. (2010). The HPV vaccination campaign: A project of moral regulation in an era of biopolitics. *Canadian Journal of Sociology*, 35(1), 63–82.

Cutts, F. T., Franceschi, S., Goldie, S., *et al.* (2007). Human papillomavirus and HPV vaccines: A review. *Bulletin of the World Health Organization*, 85(9), 649–732.

Cvetkovich, G., and Lofstedt, R. E. (1999). *Social Trust and the Management of Risk*. New York: Earthscan Publications.

Cvetkovich, G. T., and Winter, P. L. (2002). *Social Trust and the Management of Threatened and Endangered Species: A Study of Communities of Interest and Communities of Place*. Albany, CA: Pacific Southwest Research Station, Forest Service, U.S. Department of Agriculture.

Demicheli, V., Jefferson, T., Al-Ansary, L. A., *et al.* (2014). Vaccines for preventing influenza in healthy adults. *Cochrane Database of Systematic Reviews*, (3).

De Vocht, M., Claeys, A. S., Cauberghe, V., Uyttendaele, M., and Sas, B. (2016). Won't we scare them? The impact of communicating uncontrollable risks on the public's perception. *Journal of Risk Research*, 19(3), 316–330.

Dew, K. (1999). Epidemics, panic and power: representations of measles and measles vaccines. *Health*, 3(4), 379–398.

Dew, K. (2012). *The Cult and Science of Public Health: A Sociological Investigation*. New York: Berghahn Books.

Dillner, L. (2014). Is the government wrong about giving children the nasal spray flu vaccine? *The Guardian*, October 5. Available at: www.theguardian.com/lifeandstyle/2014/oct/05/government-wrong-nasal-spray-vaccine

Doshi, P. (2005). Are US flu death figures more PR than science? *BMJ*, 331(7529), 1412.

Doshi, P. (2013). Influenza: Marketing vaccine by marketing disease. *BMJ*, 346, f3037.

Dyer, O. (2015). Canadian academic's call for moratorium on HPV vaccine sparks controversy. *BMJ*, 351, h5692.

Earle, T. C., and Cvetkovich, G. (1995). *Social Trust: Toward a Cosmopolitan Society* Westport, CT: Praeger.

Einhorn, H. J., and Hogwarth, R. M. (1985). Ambiguity and uncertainty in probabilistic inference. *Psychological Review*, 92(4), 433–461.

Eisenberg, E. M. (1984). Ambiguity as strategy in organizational communication. *Communication Monographs*, 51, 227–242.

Engelhard, D. (2009). The influenza is dangerous and threatening – the vaccine is effective, safe and much recommended. November 15. Available at: www.engineers. org.il/_Uploads/6569profengelhart.pdf

European Medicines Agency. (2009). European Medicines Agency recommends authorisation of two vaccines for influenza pandemic (H1N1) 2009. Press release. September 25. London: European Medicines Agency.

European Medicines Agency. (2011). Press release: European Medicines Agency recommends restricting use of Pandemrix. July 21. Available at: www.ema.europa. eu/ema/index.jsp?curl=pages/news_and_events/news/2011/07/news_detail_001312. jspandmid=WC0b01ac058004d5c1 (accessed May 6, 2016).

Even, D., Yagna, Y., and Levi, T. (, 2009). The Ministry of Health: In the coming days more people will die from swine flu . *Ha'aretz*. July 28. Available at: www.haaretz. co.il/misc/1.1273309

Fauci, A. (2009). How safe is the Flu vaccine? YouTube. October 26. Available at: www.youtube.com/watch?v=TE4cNqcBCEQ (accessed May 6, 2016).

FDA. (1984). 21 CFR Part 630 [Docket Number 84N-0178] Additional Standards for Viral Vaccines; Poliovirus Vaccine, Live, Oral. Available at: http://dev.hisunim.org.il/ wp-content/uploads/2015/09/FDA-Any-Possible-Doubts-Cannot-Be-Allowed.pdf (accessed May 2, 2016).

Fischhoff, B. (2004). A diagnostic for risk communication failers. In W. Leiss and D. Powell (Eds.), *Mad Cows and Mother's Milk: The Perils of Poor Risk Communication* (2nd Edition, pp. 26–40). Montreal: McGill-Queen's University Press.

Foucault, M. (1972). *The Archaeology of Knowledge*. London: Tavistock Publications.

Foucault, M. (1977). *Discipline and Punish: The Birth of the Prison*. New York: Pantheon Books.

Foucault, M. (1980). *Power/Knowledge: Selected Interviews and Other Writings*. Brighton: Harvester.

Fox, T. (2009). The role of uncertainty intolerance in European risk governance. Paper presented at the Risk Research Symposium, King's College London.

France 24. (, 2009). Doctor says FLU VACCINE will cause 60,000 deaths in France alone. France 24, September 14. Available at: www.youtube.com/watch?v=dXAK_ 6iZbH0 (accessed May 6, 2016).

Frankfort, H., Frankfort, H. A., Wilson, J. A., Jacobsen, T., and Irwin, W. A. (1946). *The Intellectual Adventure of Ancient Man: An Essay on Speculative Thought in the Ancient Near East*. Chicago: The University of Chicago Press.

Frazer, J. G. (2002). *The Golden Bough: A Study in Magic and Religion* (Abridged edition). Mineola, NY: Dover.

Frewer, L., Hunt, S., Brennan, M., Kuznesof, S., Ness, M., and Ritson, C. (2003). The views of scientific experts on how the public conceptualize uncertainty. *Journal of Risk Research*, 6(1), 75–85.

Frieden, T. (2015). Keep measles out of your community . *USA TODAY*, February 22, Available at: www.usatoday.com/story/opinion/2015/02/22/cdc-tom-frieden-measles-outbreak-vaccine-column/23694391/ (accessed May 2, 2016).

Gaglani, M., Pruszynski, J., Murthy, K., *et al.* (2016). Influenza vaccine effectiveness against 2009 pandemic influenza A(H1N1) virus differed by vaccine type during 2013–2014 in the United States. *Journal of Infectious Diseases*, 213(10), 1546–1556.

GAO. (2011). Influenza Pandemic: Lessons from the H1N1 Pandemic should be incorporated into future planning. (No. GAO-11–632). Washington, DC: The Government Accountability Office.

Garcia-Berthou, E., and Alcaraz, C. (2004). Incongruence between test statistics and P values in medical papers. *BMC Medical Research Methodology*, 4, 13.

German, Y. (August 16, 2013). So why to vaccinate the children? Available at: www.facebook.com/GermanYeshAtid/posts/635167036501039?comment_id=6763998andoffset=0andtotal_comments=144 (accessed April 30, 2016).

Gesser-Edelsburg, A., and Shir-Raz, Y. (2015). Science vs. fear: The Ebola quarantine debate as a case study that reveals how the public perceives risk. *Journal of Risk Research*, 1–23. DOI: 10.1080/13669877.2015.1100659.

Gesser-Edelsburg, A., Shir-Raz, Y., Bar-Lev Sassoni, O., James, J. J., and Green, M. S. (2016). Outbreak or epidemic? How Obama's language choice transformed the Ebola outbreak into an epidemic. *Disaster Medicine and Public Health Preparedness, FirstView*, 1–5.

Gesser-Edelsburg, A., Shir-Raz, Y., and Green, M. S. (2016). Why do parents who usually vaccinate their children hesitate or refuse? General good vs. individual risk. *Journal of Risk Research*, 19(4), 405–424.

Gesser-Edelsburg, A., and Zemach, M. (2012). From a fiasco to the Supertanker grand finale: Israeli Prime Minister Netanyahu's crisis communication during the Carmel disaster. *Journal of Risk Research*, 15(8), 967–989.

GLZ. (2013). The Ministry of Health Director General: The polio vaccine is safe. Vaccinate your children. Available at: http://glz.co.il/1087-24007-he/Galatz.aspx (accessed May 6, 2016).

Godlee, F. (2012). Clinical trial data for all drugs in current use. *BMJ*, 345, e7304.

Golan, D., and Linn, S. (2015). From statistical associations to scientific causality. *Harefuah*, 154(6), 389–393, 403.

Goldacre, B. (2013). *Bad Pharma: How Drug Companies Mislead Doctors and Harm Patients*. New York: Faber and Faber.

Goldstein, M. A., Goodman, A., del Carmen, M. G., and Wilbur, D. C. (2009). Case 10–2009 – A 23-year-old woman with an abnormal papanicolaou smear. *New England Journal of Medicine*, 360(13), 1337–1344.

Goodman, S. N. (1999). Toward evidence-based medical statistics. 1: The P value fallacy. *Annals of Internal Medicine*, 130(12), 995–1004.

Grabowska, A. K., and Riemer, A. B. (2012). The invisible enemy – How human papillomaviruses avoid recognition and clearance by the host immune system. *The Open Virology Journal*, 6(Suppl 2), 249–256.

Graves, C. (2015). Why debunking myths about vaccines hasn't convinced dubious parents. *The Harvard Business Review*, February 20.

Green, M. S., Swartz, T., Mayshar, E., *et al.* (2002). When is an epidemic an epidemic? *The Israel Medical Association Journal: IMAJ*, 4(1), 3–6.

Grimaldi-Bensouda, L., Guillemot, D., Godeau, B., *et al.* (2014). Autoimmune disorders and quadrivalent human papillomavirus vaccination of young female subjects. *Journal of Internal Medicine*, 275(4), 398–408.

Halperin, E. (2009). What exactly is the Ministry of Health afraid of? *Ha'aretz*, December 29. Available at: www.haaretz.co.il/misc/1.1297208

Hathaway, J. K. (2012). HPV: Diagnosis, prevention, and treatment. *Clinical Obstetrics and Gynecology*, 55(3), 671–680.

Heier, M. S., Gautvik, K. M., Wannag, E., *et al.* (2013). Incidence of narcolepsy in Norwegian children and adolescents after vaccination against H1N1 influenza A. *Sleep Medicine*, 14(9), 867–871.

Hilgartner, S. (1992). The social construction of risk objects: Or, how to pry open networks of risk. In J. F. Short and L. Clarek (Eds.), *Organizations, Uncertainties, and Risk* (pp. 39–53). Boulder, CO: Westview Press.

Horne, Z., Powell, D., Hummel, J. E., and Holyoak, K. J. (2015). Countering anti-vaccination attitudes. *Proceedings of the National Academy of Sciences of the United States of America*, 112(33), 10321–10324.

Horton, M. (2010). Common myths about vaccines debunked. September 13. Sacramento: California Department of Public Health.

House of Commons Committee of Public Accounts. (2014). Access to clinical trial information and the stockpiling of Tamiflu. London: TSO.

Ioannidis, J. P. A. (2005). Why most published research findings are false. *PLoS Med*, 2(8), e124.

Jefferson, T., Di Pietrantonj, C., Al-Ansary, L. A., *et al.* (2010). Vaccines for preventing influenza in the elderly. *Cochrane Database of Systematic Reviews*, 17(2).

Jefferson, T., Di Pietrantonj, C., Rivetti, A., *et al.* (2010). Vaccines for preventing influenza in healthy adults. *Cochrane Database of Systematic Reviews*, 7.

Jefferson, T., Jones, M. A., Doshi, P., et al. (2014). Neuraminidase inhibitors for preventing and treating influenza in adults and children. *Cochrane Database of Systematic Reviews*, 4.

Jeffrey, S. (2009). AAN 2009: No increase in Guillain-Barré after HPV vaccination, but further monitoring warranted. Available at: www.medscape.com/viewarticle/ 588510 (accessed May 6, 2016).

Jemal, A., Center, M. M., DeSantis, C., and Ward, E. M. (2010). Global patterns of cancer incidence and mortality rates and trends. *Cancer Epidemiology Biomarkers and Prevention*, 19(8), 1893–1907.

Jeng, M. (2006). Error in statistical tests of error in statistical tests. *BMC Medical Research Methodology*, 6, 45.

Kahneman, D., Slovic, P., and Tversky, A. (1982). *Judgment Under Uncertainty: Heuristics and Biases*. Cambridge: Cambridge University Press.

Kaliner, E., Kopel, E., Anis, E., et al. (2015). The Israeli public health response to wild poliovirus importation. *The Lancet Infectious Diseases*, 15(10), 1236–1242.

Klinke, A., and Renn, O. (2002). A new approach to risk evaluation and management: Risk-based, precaution-based, and discourse-based strategies. *Risk Analysis*, 22(6), 1071–1094.

Laine, C., Horton, R., DeAngelis, C. D., *et al.* (2007). Clinical trial registration. *BMJ*, 334(7605), 1177–1178.

Laino, C. (2009). Gardasil linked to nerve disorder: Cervical cancer vaccine may raise risk of Guillain-Barré syndrome. WebMD, April 30. Available at: www.webmd.com/ cancer/cervical-cancer/news/20090430/gardasil-linked-to-nerve-disorder

Little, D. T., and Ward, H. R. G. (2012). Premature ovarian failure 3 years after menarche in a 16-year-old girl following human papillomavirus vaccination. *BMJ Case Reports*, 2012. doi:10.1136/bcr-2012-006879.

Little, D. T., and Ward, H. R. G. (2014). Adolescent premature ovarian insufficiency following Human Papillomavirus Vaccination: A case series seen in general practice. *Journal of Investigative Medicine High Impact Case Reports*, 2(4). doi: 10.1177/2324709614556129.

Lofstedt, R. E. (2005). *Risk Management in Post-Trust Societies*. London: Palgrave Macmillan.

Lofstedt, R. E. (2006). How can we make food risk communication better?: Where are we and where are we going? *Journal of Risk Research*, 9(8), 869–890.

Lowy, I. (2011). *A Woman's Disease: The History of Cervical Cancer*. Oxford: Oxford University Press.

Lule, J. (2001). *Daily News, Eternal Stories: The Mythological Role of Journalism*. New York: The Guilford Press.

Macera, C. A., Shaffer, R. A., and Shaffer, P. M. (2013). *Introduction to Epidemiology: Distribution and Determinants of Disease Humans (Public Health Basics)*. Clifton Park, NY: Delmar, Cengage Learning.

Malinowski, B. (2014). *Magic, Science and Religion and Other Essays*. Sparks, MD: McCormick Press.

Martínez-Lavín, M., Martínez-Martínez, L. A., and Reyes-Loyola, P. (2015). HPV vaccination syndrome. A questionnaire-based study. *Clinical Rheumatology*, 34(11), 1981–1983.

Martuzzi, M., and Ticknet, J. A. (2004). *The Precautionary Principle: Protecting Public Health, the Environment and the Future of Our Children*. Copenhagen: World Health Organization.

Matheson, A. (2008). Corporate science and the husbandry of scientific and medical knowledge by the pharmaceutical industry. *BioSocieties*, 3(04), 355–382.

Matzliah, R. (2013). Health Minister: Thousands of people infected with polio in the south, the disease may return. Available at: www.mako.co.il/news-israel/health/Article-d5976e762d86041004.htm (accessed April 30, 2016).

Maurice, J.Measles outbreak in DR Congo an "epidemic emergency". *The Lancet*, 386 (9997), 943.

McCafferty, L. A. E. (2006). Editorial: HPV awareness. *ADVANCE for Nurses*, 6(12), 5.

McComas, K. A., and Trumbo, C. W. (2001). Source credibility in environmental health-risk controversies: Application of Meyer's credibility index. *Risk Analysis*, 21(3), 467–480.

McElduff, P., Attia, J., Ewald, B., Cockburn, J., and Heller, R. (2002). Estimating the contribution of individual risk factors to disease in a person with more than one risk factor. *Journal of Clinical Epidemiology*, 55(6), 588–592.

Medical Products Agency. (2010). The MPA investigates reports of narcolepsy in patients vaccinated with Pandemrix. Uppsala: Lakemedelsverket.

Medical Products Agency. (2011). Report from an epidemiological study in Sweden on vaccination with Pandemrix and narcolepsy. Available at: https://lakemedelsverket.se/english/All-news/NYHETER-2011/Report-from-an-epidemiological-study-in-Sweden-on-vaccination-with-Pandemrix-and-narcolepsy-/ (accessed May 6, 2016).

Michaels, D. (2008). *Doubt Is Their Product: How Industry's Assault on Science Threatens Your Health*. Oxford: Oxford University Press.

Miller, E., Andrews, N., Stellitano, L., Stowe, J., Winstone, A. M., Shneerson, J. et al. (2013). Risk of narcolepsy in children and young people receiving AS03 adjuvanted pandemic A/H1N1 2009 influenza vaccine: retrospective analysis. *BMJ*, 346, f794.

Ministry of Health Israel. (2008). A summary of the advisory committee on infectious diseases and immunization meeting in 17.2.08 on conditioning the entrance to the education system upon the presentation of a confirmation of receiving vaccines. Available at: www.health.gov.il/Services/Committee/IDAC/Documents/CMV170220 08.pdf (accessed May 6, 2016).

Ministry of Health Israel. (2011). A summary of the Israeli advisory committee on infectious diseases and immunization meeting in 11.8.11 on the presentation of vaccines' side effects in the Ministry of Health publications. Available at: www.hea lth.gov.il/Services/Committee/IDAC/Documents/CMV11082011.pdf (accessed May 6, 2016).

Ministry of Health Israel. (2013a). A poliovirus has been exposed in Rahat settlements' sewage system. (May 28, 2013 update). Available at: www.health.gov.il

Ministry of Health Israel. (2013b). A poliovirus has been exposed also in Kiryat Gat and Ashdod sewage system. June 12. Available at: www.health.gov.il/News AndEvents/SpokemanMesseges/Pages/13062013_1.aspx

Ministry of Health Israel. (2013c). Just two drops, and the family is protected from the risk of polio. August 4. Available at: www.health.gov.il/English/Topics/Vaccination/ two_drops/Pages/default.aspx (accessed May 2, 2016).

Ministry of Health Israel. (2013d). Polio update (August 18, 2013 update). Available at: www.health.gov.il/English/News_and_Events/Spokespersons_Messages/Pages/180820 13_2.aspx

Ministry of Health Israel. (2013e). Polio update – A poliovirus also in Ofakim. August 21. Available at: www.health.gov.il/NewsAndEvents/SpokemanMesseges/Pages/21032013_ 5.aspx

Ministry of Health Israel. (2013f). A poliovirus has been exposed in Iron's sewage treatment plant. August 27. Available at: www.health.gov.il/NewsAndEvents/Sp okemanMesseges/Pages/27082013_1.aspx

Ministry of Health Israel. (2013g). A poliovirus has been exposed in Jerusalem's sewage treatment plant. September 9. Available at: www.health.gov.il/News AndEvents/SpokemanMesseges/Pages/09092013_2.aspx

Ministry of Health Israel. (2015). A summary of the advisory committee on infectious diseases and immunization meeting in 19.8.15 on winter flu vaccination. August 27. Available at: www.health.gov.il/Services/Committee/IDAC/Documents/CMV19082015. pdf (accessed May 6, 2016).

Moynihan, R., and Cassels, A. (2005). *Selling Sickness*. New York: Nation Books.

Naim, M. (2009). The Ministry of Health responds with rage: False publications in the media regarding swine flu vaccinations. *Kan-naim*, November 10. Available at: www.kanisrael.co.il/artical.asp?id=15077andcid=809

National Advisory Committee on Immunization. (2007). Statement on human papillomavirus vaccine. *Canada Communicable Disease Report*, 33(ACS-2).

National Narcolepsy Study Steering Committee. (2012). *Investigation of an Increase in the Incidence of Narcolepsy in children and Adolescents in 2009 and 2010*. Available at: www.thehealthwell.info/node/773852

National Women's Health Network. (2015). Cervical cancer prevention and screening. Available at: www.nwhn.org/cervical-cancer-prevention-and-screening/ (accessed May 2, 2016).

NHS. (2016). Vaccinations: Vaccine myths. Available at: www.nhs.uk/conditions/va ccinations/pages/myths-truths-kids-vaccines.aspx (accessed April 28, 2016).

NIH. (2015). *Human Papillomavirus (HPV) Vaccines.* Bethesda, MD: National Cancer Institute.

Nohynek, H., Jokinen, J., Partinen, M., *et al.* (2012). AS03 adjuvanted AH1N1 vaccine associated with an abrupt increase in the incidence of childhood narcolepsy in Finland. *PLoS ONE*, 7(3), e33536.

Nowak, G. (2004). Planning for the 2004–2005 influenza vaccination season: A communication situation analysis. Available at: www.fisique.ca/documents/CDC_2004_ flu_nowak.pdf (accessed May 1, 2016).

Nowotny, H., Scott, P., and Gibbons, M. (2001). *Re-Thinking Science: Knowledge and the Public in an Age of Uncertainty.* Cambridge: Polity Press in association with Blackwell Publishers.

Nyhan, B., and Reifler, J. (2015). Does correcting myths about the flu vaccine work? An experimental evaluation of the effects of corrective information. *Vaccine*, 33(3), 459–464.

Nyhan, B., Reifler, J., Richey, S., and Freed, G. L. (2014). Effective messages in vaccine promotion: A randomized trial. *Pediatrics*, 133(4), e835–e842.

Osterholm, M. T., Kelley, N. S., Sommer, A., and Belongia, E. A. (2012). Efficacy and effectiveness of influenza vaccines: A systematic review and meta-analysis. *The Lancet Infectious Diseases*, 12(1), 36–44.

Palenchar, M. J., and Heath, R. L. (2002). Another part of the risk communication model: Analysis of communication processes and message content. *Journal of Public Relations Research*, 14(2), 127–158.

Panel of Independent Experts. (2015). *Report of the Ebola Interim Assessment Panel.* Geneva: World Health Organization.

Parkin, D. M. (2006). The global health burden of infection-associated cancers in the year 2002. *International Journal of Cancer*, 118(12), 3030–3044.

Parsons, P. J. (2007). Integrating ethics with strategy: Analyzing disease-branding. *Corporate Communications: An International Journal*, 12(3), 267–279.

Payer, L. (1992). *Disease-Mongers: How Doctors, Drug Companies, and Insurers Are Making You Feel Sick.* New York: John Wiley & Sons, Inc.

Pellegrino, P., Carnovale, C., Pozzi, M., et al. (2014). On the relationship between human papilloma virus vaccine and autoimmune diseases. *Autoimmunity Reviews*, 13(7), 736–741.

Persson, I., Granath, F., Askling, J., Ludvigsson, J. F., Olsson, T., and Feltelius, N. (2014). Risks of neurological and immune-related diseases, including narcolepsy, after vaccination with Pandemrix: a population- and registry-based cohort study with over 2 years of follow-up. *Journal of Internal Medicine*, 275(2), 172–190.

Petersen, A., and Lupton, D. (1996). *The New Public Health: Health and Self in the Age of Risk.* St Leonards, NSW: Allen and Unwin.

Ponsford, D. (2016). NRS: Daily Mail most popular UK newspaper in print and online with 23m readers a month. *Press Gazette*, February 26. Available at: www. pressgazette.co.uk/nrs-daily-mail-most-popular-uk-newspaper-print-and-online-23m-readers-month-0

Poortinga, W., and Pidgeon, N. F. (2005). Trust in risk regulation: Cause or consequence of the acceptability of GM food? *Risk Analysis*, 25(1), 199–209.

Popper, K. (2002). *Conjectures and Refutations: The Growth of Scientific Knowledge* (2nd edition). London: Routledge.

Prayle, A. P., Hurley, M. N., and Smyth, A. R. (2012). Compliance with mandatory reporting of clinical trial results on ClinicalTrials.gov: Cross sectional study. *BMJ*, 344, d7373.

Press TV. (2009). Many Italian physicians reject swine flu vaccine! Available at: Socio-Economics History Blog (accessed November 9).

PreventDisease. (2009). Canada sets aside 170,000 doses of the Arepanrix H1N1 vaccine after reactions. Available at: www.Preventdisease.com. November 20.

Proctor, R. N. (2012). *Golden Holocaust: Origins of the Cigarette Catastrophe and the Case for Abolition*. Berkeley: University of California Press.

PublicHealth. (2016). Understating vaccines: Vaccine myths debunked. Available at: www.PublicHealth.org

Ravetz, J. R. (2001). Models of risk: an exploration. In M. Hisschemöller, R. Hoppe, W. N. Dunn and J. R. Ravetz (Eds.), *Knowledge, Power, and Participation in Environmental Policy Analysis* (pp. 471–491). New Brunswick, NJ: Transaction Publishers.

Renn, O. (2006). Risk governance: Towards an integrative approach. IRGC White Paper No 1. Available at: www.irgc.org/IMG/pdf/IRGC_WP_No_1_Risk_Governa nce__reprinted_version_.pdf (accessed April 29, 2016).

Renn, O., and Walker, K. (2008). *Global Risk Governance: Concept and Practice Using the IRGC Framework*. Dordrecht: Springer Netherlands.

Richman, A. (2005). Human papillomavirus: a catalyst to a killer. *American Journal of Health Education*, 36(3), 166–173.

Rosenbaum, L. (2015). Communicating uncertainty – Ebola, public health, and the scientific process. *The New England Journal of Medicine*, 372(1), 7–9.

Rothman, K. J., and Greenland, S. (2002). Causation and causal inference. In R. Detels, J. McEwen, R. Beaglehole and H. Tanaka (Eds.), *Oxford Textbook of Public Health: The Scope of Public Health* (4th Edition, pp. 641–654). Oxford: Oxford University Press.

Rothman, K. J., and Greenland, S. (2005). Causation and causal inference in epidemiology. *American Journal of Public Health*, 95(S1), S144–S150.

Sandman, P. (1989). Hazard versus outrage in the public perception of risk. In V. T. Covello, D. B. McCallum and M. T. Pavlove (Eds.), *Effective Risk Communication: The Role and Responsibility of Government and Nongovernment Organizations* (pp. 45–49). New York: Plenum Press.

Sandman, P. (2003). Four kinds of risk communication. *The Synergist (Journal of the American Industrial Hygiene Association)*, April 26–27.

Sandman, P., and Lanard, J. (2011). Explaining and proclaiming uncertainty: Risk communication lessons from Germany's E. coli outbreak. Available at: www.psa ndman.com/col/GermanEcoli.htm (accessed November 23, 2014).

Scheller, N. M., Svanström, H., Pasternak, B., et al. (2015). Quadrivalent HPV vacci-nation and risk of multiple sclerosis and other demyelinating diseases of the central nervous system. *JAMA*, 313(1), 54–61.

Schiffman, M., and Kjaer, S. K. (2003). Natural history of anogenital human papillomavirus infection and neoplasia. *JNCI Monographs*, 2003(31), 14–19.

Segal, R. A. (2004). *Myth: A Very Short Introduction*. Oxford: Oxford University Press.

Shafran-Gittelman, I. (2013). Why I haven't vaccinated my children yet. *Haaretz*, August 22. Available at: www.haaretz.co.il/opinions/1.2103948

Shir-Raz, Y. (2014). *Under the Regulation Radar: Strategies and Tactics of Pharmaceutical Companies to Promote Drugs and Medical Products in Israel*. Haifa: University of Haifa.

Shrader-Frechette, K. (1996). Methodological rules for four classes of scientific uncertainty. In J. Lemons (Ed.), *Scientific Uncertainty and Environmental Problem Solving* (pp. 12–39). Malden, MA: Blackwell Science.

Siegrist, M., Cvetkovich, G., and Roth, C. (2000). Salient value similarity, social trust, and risk/benefit perception. *Risk Analysis*, 20(3), 353–362.

Siegrist, M., Gutscher, H., and Earle, T. C. (2005). Perception of risk: The influence of general trust, and general confidence. *Journal of Risk Research*, 8(2), 145–156.

Simmons, J. P., Nelson, L. D., and Simonsohn, U. (2011). False-positive psychology: Undisclosed flexibility in data collection and analysis allows presenting anything as significant. *Psychological Science*, 22(11), 1359–1366.

Sloane, M. (2014). This year's flu vaccine less effective than hoped. Available at: www.webmd.com/cold-and-flu/news/20141204/this-years-flu-vaccine-less-effective-than-hoped (accessed May 6, 2016).

Slovic, P. (1991). Beyond numbers: A broader perspective on risk perception and risk communication. In D. G. Mayo and R. D. Hollander (Eds.), *Acceptable Evidence: Science and Values in Risk Management* (pp. 48–65). New York: Oxford University Press.

Slovic, P. (1995). The construction of preference. *American Psychologist*, 50(5), 364–371.

Slovic, P. (1999). Trust, emotion, sex, politics, and science: Surveying the risk-assessment battlefield. *Risk Analysis*, 19(4), 689–701.

Slovic, P., Finucane, M., Peters, E., and MacGregor, D. (2004). Risk as analysis and risk as feelings: Some thoughts about affect, reason, risk and rationality. *Risk Analysis*, 24(2), 311–322.

Smith, G. D., and Ebrahim, S. (2002). Data dredging, bias, or confounding: They can all get you into the BMJ and the Friday papers. *BMJ*, 325(7378), 1437–1438.

Social Health and Family Affairs Committee (2010). The handling of the H1N1 pandemic: More transparency needed. *Doc. 12283* (Vol. 12). (Rapporteur: Mr. Paul Flynn). Strasbourg: Parliamentary Assembly of the Council of Europe.

Souayah, N., Michas-Martin, P. A., Nasar, A., *et al.* (2011). Guillain-Barré syndrome after Gardasil vaccination: Data from Vaccine Adverse Event Reporting System 2006–2009. *Vaccine*, 29(5), 886–889.

Spencer, J. (2007). *Cervical Cancer*. New York: Chelsea House Publications.

Stafford, N. (2009). Only 12% of Germans say they will have H1N1 vaccine after row blows up over safety of adjuvants. *BMJ*, 339, b4335.

Stern, D. J. (2009). Letter to Professor Engelhard of the Ministry of Health, Israel. November 4. Available at: http://israeltruthtimes.blogspot.co.il/2009/11/this-is-letter-that-i-will-be-sending.html (accessed May 6, 2016).

Sterne, J. A. C., and Smith, G. D. (2001). Sifting the evidence – what's wrong with significance tests? *Physical Therapy*, 81(8), 1464–1469.

Susser, M. (1977). Judgement and causal inference: criteria in epidemiologic studies. *American Journal of Epidemiology*, 105(1), 1–15.

Talmor, N. (2009). Fell from a scaffolding and declared dead from swine flu. *Walla! News*. October 26. Available at: http://news.walla.co.il/item/1596185

The Alpha-Tocopherol Beta Carotene Cancer Prevention Study Group. (1994). The effect of vitamin E and Beta Carotene on the incidence of lung cancer and other cancers in male smokers. *New England Journal of Medicine*, 330, 1029–1035.

The Cochrane Collaboration. (2014). Tamiflu and Relenza: How effective are they? The BMJ and Cochrane call on government and health policy decision makers to review guidance on use of Tamiflu in light of most recent evidence. April 10. Available at: http://community.cochrane.org/features/tamiflu-relenza-how-effective-are-they

The Committee for the Advancement of Woman Status. (2007). *Protocol No. 55 from The Committee for the Advancement of Woman Status.* May 21. Available at: www.knesset.gov.il/protocols/data/rtf/maamad/2007-05-21.rtf

The Hindu Business Line. (2015). Public health activists oppose move to introduce HPV vaccine in universal immunisation. Available at: www.thehindubusinessline.com/news/public-health-activists-oppose-move-to-introduce-hpv-vaccine-in-universal-immunisation/article7518942.ece

Thompson, P., and Dean, W. (1996). Competing conceptions of risk. *Risk, Health, Safety and Environment,* 7(136).

TIRC. (1964). *Reports on Tobacco and Health Research, Winter 1964–1965.* Washington, DC: Tobacco Institute Inc.

Tomljenovic, L., Colafrancesco, S., Perricone, C., and Shoenfeld, Y. (2014). Postural Orthostatic Tachycardia with chronic fatigue after HPV vaccination as part of the "autoimmune/auto-inflammatory syndrome induced by adjuvants": Case report and literature review. *Journal of Investigative Medicine High Impact Case Reports,* 2(1).

Tomljenovic, L., and Shaw, C. A. (2013). Human papillomavirus (HPV) vaccine policy and evidence-based medicine: Are they at odds? *Annals of Medicine,* 45(2), 182–193.

Trafimow, D., and Marks, M. (2015). Editorial. *Basic and Applied Social Psychology,* 37(1), 1–2.

Turner, E. H., Matthews, A. M., Linardatos, E., Tell, R. A., and Rosenthal, R. (2008). Selective publication of antidepressant trials and its influence on apparent efficacy. *New England Journal of Medicine,* 358(3), 252–260.

Tylor, E. B. (1920). *Primitive Culture: Research into the Development of Mythology, Philosophy, Religion, Language, Art, and Custom.* London: John Murray.

Ulmer, R. R., and Sellnow, T. L. (1997). Strategic ambiguity and the ethic of significant choice in the tobacco industry's crisis communication. *Communication Studies,* 48(3), 215–233.

Vaarala, O., Vuorela, A., Partinen, M., Baumann, M., Freitag, T. L., Meri, S. *et al.* (2014). Antigenic differences between AS03 adjuvanted influenza A (H1N1) pandemic vaccines: Implications for Pandemrix-associated narcolepsy risk. *PLoS ONE,* 9(12), e114361.

van Asselt, M. B. A., and Vos, E. (2005). The precautionary principle in times of intermingled uncertainty and risk: some regulatory complexities. *Water Science and Technology,* 52(6), 35–41.

van Asselt, M. B. A., and Vos, E. (2006). The precautionary principle and the uncertainty paradox. *Journal of Risk Research,* 9(4), 313–336.

van Asselt, M. B. A., and Vos, E. (2008). Wrestling with uncertain risks: EU regulation of GMOs and the uncertainty paradox. *Journal of Risk Research,* 11(1–2), 281–300.

van Asselt, M. B. A., Vos, E., and Rooijackers, B. (2009). Science, knowledge and uncertainty in EU risk regulation. In M. Everson and E. Vos (Eds.), *Uncertain Risks Regulated* (pp. 359–388). London: Routledge-Cavendish.

Vlaeyen, J. (2008). Onzekerheid maakt mensen bang. In J. P. M. Geraets, M. B. A. van Asselt and L. Koenen (Eds.), *Leven met Onzekerheid Stichting* (pp. 16–18). Den Haag: Bio-Wetenschappen en Maatschappij.

Wallsten, T. S. (1990). The costs and benefits of vague information. In R. Hogarth (Ed.), *Insights in Decision Making. A Tribute to the Late Hillel Einhorn* (pp. 28–43). Chicago: University of Chicago Press.

Wertheim, D. (2014). TGI Survey for the first half of 2014: The gap between Israel Today and Yedioth Ahronoth is expanding. *Walla*, July 28. Available at: http://b.walla.co.il/item/2769911

WHO. (2010). Transcript of virtual press conference with Dr Margaret Chan, Director-General, World Health Organization and Dr Keiji Fukuda, Special Adviser to the Director-General on Pandemic Influenza. August 10. Geneva: World Health Organization.

WHO. (2013a). *HPV Vaccine Communication: Special Considerations for a Unique Vaccine*. Geneva: World Health Organization.

WHO. (2013b). *Chapter 4: HPV Vaccination: Comprehensive Cervical Cancer Control: A Guide to Essential Practice (C4 GEP)*. Geneva: World Health Organization.

WHO. (2015). Human papillomavirus (HPV) and cervical cancer. Fact sheet N° 380. Available at: www.who.int/mediacentre/factsheets/fs380/en/ (accessed May 1, 2016).

WHO. (2016a). *Six Common Misconceptions about Immunization*. Geneva: World Health Organization.

WHO. (2016b). What are some of the myths – and facts – about vaccination? Online Q&A. Available at: www.who.int/features/qa/84/en/ (accessed April 28, 2016).

Woolston, C. (2015). Psychology journal bans P values: Test for reliability of results 'too easy to pass', say editors. *Nature*, 519(7541), 9.

Wynne, B. (1992). Uncertainty and environmental learning: Reconceiving science and policy in the preventive paradigm. *Global Environmental Change*, 2(2), 111–127.

Wynne, B. (1995). Technology assessment and reflexive social learning: Observations from the risk field. In A. Rip, T. J. Misa and J. W. Schot (Eds.), *Managing Technology in Society: The Approach of Constructive Technology Assessment* (pp. 19–37). London: Pinter Publishers.

Wynne, B. (2001). Creating public alienation: Expert cultures of risk and ethics on GMOs. *Science as Culture*, 10(4), 445–481.

Yaphe, J., Edman, R., Knishkowy, B., and Herman, J. (2001). The association between funding by commercial interests and study outcome in randomized controlled drug trials. *Family Practice*, 18(6), 565–568.

# 5    The Role of Medical Experts and Health Journalists

Journalists and doctors are often described as two very different kinds of professionals, who draw from different disciplines and spheres of discourse. They have different values and goals, as well as different concepts of validity, objectivity, and significance (Leask et al., 2010). Yet in fact, these two professions have much in common. First and foremost, both journalists and doctors are the main channels for funneling health information to the public, which is especially critical in the periods preceding and following epidemics. Both doctors and journalists mediate between the organizations and governments and the public. In the technological reality of citizen journalism and participatory journalism, the role of journalists has transformed from the traditional media, which raises many questions and challenges regarding the nature of their role. However, as long as journalists carry out a professional role, their job is to voice the public's concerns. Doctors mediate as well, but while journalists are considered outsider influential stakeholders, public health workers are expected to operate as the organizations' voice. These similarities and differences underlie the ethical and communication questions raised in the present chapter. Above the doctors and the journalists looms the pharmaceutical industry as a major stakeholder that holds excessive influence in the field of risk communication. This chapter treats the industry's role, and to what extent it affects or manipulates doctors and journalists.

## Part 1: How do journalists write about health in a reality of uncertainty?

In the complex and fast-changing reality of the 21st century, with unpredictable epidemics that are often affected by social, political, ethnic, and genetic factors, emerging health crises often entail a significant dimension of scientific uncertainty. One of the challenges facing health journalists is how to communicate issues of uncertainty in the media. Journalists are constantly faced with the need to report debatable issues, such as the advisability of seasonal flu vaccines and modes of virus contagion (for example, whether the Ebola virus spreads through bodily fluids or via air). Researchers who examined the representation of scientific uncertainty in journalism concerning subjects such as climate change and biotechnological research have noted a number of contradictory approaches, which point to the various considerations and interests of individual journalists and news organizations. Stocking and Holstein (1993) call these interests "socially constructed."

### Constructing the reality of diseases and medicines

The theory of social construction of reality describes the media's role in constructing a symbolic reality, different from the "real" one (Gerbner, 1969). According to the theory, the mass media serve as mediators, although their role is often invisible, in our daily lives (Morgan and Signorielli, 1990), and shape our perceptions of the world and understanding of reality (Shoemaker and Reese, 1996). Yet, the media are far from being a neutral mediator. In fact, the lens through which they present images subtly emphasizes the perspective of elites and social interest groups, including economic and political groups (Gamson, 1992; Gans, 1979).

In the spirit of the social construction of reality theory, many studies have examined media representation of diseases, and pointed to the tendency of presenting a reality that is significantly different from the real one, i.e., the official data. This tendency is reflected, among other things, in significant gaps in the coverage of various diseases and their actual proportions in the population, as well as in the mortality rates and the economic burden these diseases pose (Bomlitz and Brezis, 2008; Hoffman-Goetz and MacDonald, 1999; Weimann and Lev, 2006). For example, Bomlitz and Brezis (2008) investigated the relationship between causes of death in the USA in 2003 and media coverage. They counted mass media reports in the United States on emerging and chronic health hazards (Severe Acute Respiratory Syndrome (SARS), bioterrorism, West Nile Fever, AIDS, smoking and physical inactivity) for the year 2003, using the LexisNexis database. They found that the number of media reports inversely correlated with the actual number of deaths for the health risks evaluated. In other words, SARS and bioterrorism killed less than a dozen people in 2003, but together generated over 100,000 media reports, far more than those covering smoking and physical inactivity, which killed nearly one million Americans.

Significant gaps in the presentation of reality are also reflected in the way drugs and medical treatments are conveyed by the media. Schwitzer (2008) argues that in an era when the media themselves reported on substantial side effects and risks found with some drugs and treatments, including the Viox, coronary stents, or hormone replacement therapy, still, many of them fail to adequately quantify these risks and benefits of the products they report on.

Indeed, numerous studies have found media coverage of medicines and medical treatments suffers from many problems. These problems are manifested primarily in the tendency to cover drugs and medical technologies in a sensational and overly enthusiastic manner, giving excessive emphasis to their benefits while ignoring or hardly mentioning the risks, side effects and costs (Bubela and Caulfield, 2004; Høye and Hjortdahl, 2002; Moynihan et al.,

2000; Ransohoff and Ransohoff, 2001; Shuchman and Wilkes, 1997), as well as the limitations of scientific studies advocating the efficacy of these drugs, for instance, a tiny number of participants in a clinical study (Johnson, 1998). As Schwitzer argues:

> It is understandable that US newspapers and television stations would be interested in a story about a new drug for the common cold. Americans have one billion cold infections each year, losing millions of days of work or school. What is difficult to understand is why and how so many journalists became cheerleaders for an investigational drug that, in the end, failed to pass the test of clinical trials.
>
> (2003, p. 1403)

For example, Høye and Hjortdahl (2002) found that 79% out of 357 articles in the Norwegian media describing the benefits of new medicines failed to report on these benefits in detail; 51% presented medicines in a positive light and 19% even used overly enthusiastic terms, such as "wonder drug," and 61% of the articles did not mention potential risks involved with these drugs; and 73% did not mention costs.

Another problem several scholars warned about is the fact that journalists often fail to describe the research methods and the limitations, the funding sources supporting the research, or financial conflicts of interests of investigators, and other sources they interview (Caulfield, 2004; Kua et al., 2004; Moynihan and Sweet, 2000; Winsten, 1985). In order to be able to make informed health decisions, the audience must receive information regarding such potential conflicting interests (Shuchman and Wilkes, 1997). Reporting study limitations, funding sources and financial ties are of great importance, due to potential conflicts of interest (Cook et al., 2007). Many scholars agree that financial conflicts of interest, which unfortunately are increasing in prevalence and magnitude (Boyd and Bero, 2000; Boyd et al., 2003) have an erosive effect on the public's trust in scientists and in science (Cook et al., 2007; Drazen and Koski, 2000; Friedman, 2002). In the USA, the Statement of Principles of the Association of Health Care Journalists calls on journalists to disclose relevant conflicts of interests in their sources "as a routine part" of their work (Schwitzer, 2008). Yet, it seems that more often than not, journalists do not report such conflicts of interest (Moynihan et al., 2000; Schwitzer, 2008; Shuchman and Wilkes, 1997).

It is thus not surprising that in the conclusion of their findings, Iaboli, Caselli, Filice, Russi, and Belletti (2010) speculate "whether popular media is detrimental rather than useful to public health."

### Personal stories, sensations and scandals

Journalists occupy a midway position between healthcare professionals and creative artists. Ideally (although not actually always the case), healthcare professionals are concerned with facts and accuracy, whereas artists are interested in drama, a good story and arousing the audience's emotions. Journalists who write about health and science have to combine both approaches and present facts while conceiving an attractive story.

In this duality, which poses a formidable journalistic challenge, health reporters often opt for the sensational and attractive over depth and facts (Berzis, 2002; Nelkin, 1996). As a result, they prefer stories with dramatic results – full recovery or death, over a realistic representation of the contents (Diem et al., 1996), and emphasize aberrant findings, scandals and personal stories (Stryker et al., 2005). A compelling personal story thus becomes prominent, often at the expense of facts and the uncertain dimensions of the issue in case. Placing the patient's personal story at the center of the press report, in order to elicit readers' empathy and identification and stimulate their tear glands, often comes at the detriment of a deeper discourse.

The use of stories to illustrate news topics and turn them into more personal is considered a cornerstone in the media coverage of health issues, and particularly in the coverage of diseases and drugs (Wilson et al., 2008). For example, during the polio epidemic in the mid-20th century, along with scientific information, the American media were flooded with exciting personal stories about people suffering from the disease (Cunningham and Boom, 2013). Similarly, it was found that the media coverage of AIDS in the Israeli media was saturated with narratives and myths, and included many compelling stories (Klein, 2008). Other cases in point concern women afflicted with cervical cancer because they had not been vaccinated (Innes, 2013; Parry, 2014), or a shocking story of the death of America's first Ebola victim in 2014 (Allen and Alexander, 2014; Fantz, 2014).

Abramson (2008) describes the use of emotional stories as one aspect of a common narrative employed by health journalists when covering new drugs and medical technologies – "the good news narrative." Using this narrative, a particular health problem is described in the news article, and in order to make the audience identify with that problem, a compelling personal story of a patient suffering from it is presented. In addition, an expert is interviewed, explaining in a simple manner why the new drug or procedure is a breakthrough. Eventually, the story summarizes to what extent the patients can benefit from this new discovery. The "good news" narrative provides confirmation of our fundamental belief that medical science has advanced in its war against suffering and death (Abramson, 2008). This idealization of science and scientists is described by Rorty, who claims that the secular culture worships scientists as if they were "the priests of our time" (Rorty, 1991, pp. 35–37).

Yet, as Tversky and Kahneman (1981) have propounded, human decision-making is often guided by feelings and emotions, which are subject to inherent biases that influence and disrupt our "rational thinking." Slovic, Finucane, Peters, and MacGregor (2004) emphasized the heuristic affect in decision-making concerning risks. People consciously or unconsciously judge issues in terms of how they feel about them. Therefore, the emotional dimension emphasized by the media through heartbreaking stories reinforces people's natural biases and the tendency to make irrational decisions in conditions of uncertainty.

Furthermore, from the perspective of critical approaches in the study of discourse, incorporating literary elements in journalistic texts helps create social and political control (Bakhtin, 1981; Dew, 2012; Fairclough, 1989). The stories combined in the texts help organize the news stories into structured arguments. Thus, a consensus is built, which turns the news to a standard and accepted assertion that serves the dominant ideology.

### The sound of science

Dew argues that "as a general rule, the media take a passive attitude to information produced and disseminated by established medical and public health institutions" (1999, p. 383). Indeed, it was found that health journalists often depend on scientists, medical professionals and academic centers as sources (Lariscy et al., 2010; Len-Ríos et al., 2009), and are more likely to cite mainstream scientific sources, over sources with conflicting opinions (Pfund and Hofstadter, 1981). Moreover, in situations where journalists do not have the knowledge base to scrutinize the information they receive, their dependency on experts, especially state-supported ones, grows even further (Herman and Chomsky, 1988). In fact, their dependency on those sources is so high, that it increases their tendency to avoid controversy that might alienate those sources (Corbett and Mori, 1999). Therefore, findings from elite health sources are seldom challenged (Obregon and Waisbord, 2012). Indeed, although the coverage of scientific controversies has increased over the past decades, it was found that science and biomedical reporters are still less likely than general assignment reporters to report them (Cole, 1975). Even when they do report such controversies, they tend to prefer supportive mainstream scientific sources over alternative opinions (Pfund and Hofstadter, 1981), and present their views on those controversies as "the sound of science," making almost no attempt to question or challenge them (Dew, 1999). Not surprisingly as Corbett and Mori have concluded, "health coverage strongly resembles the priority of the medical community" (1999, p. 231). For example, Fisher, Gandy, and Janus (1981), as reported by Corbett and Mori (1999), found similarities during a 15-year period in peaks of media coverage about heart disease and peaks in the budget of the National Heart and Lung Institute. Moreover, Sumner et al. (2014) found that exaggeration in health and biomedical news is strongly associated with exaggeration in press releases issued by leading academic institutions in the UK. This means that even when the ideas and information suggested by the medical community are exaggerated or distorted, they are likely to be reproduced by the media. Thus, media coverage of health issues implies "support for the scientific and political agenda of the nation's health care delivery system" (Logan, 1991, p. 45), and the dominant ideas of the health system are the ones that prevail in the health information presented by most media outlets, and the only side of the story the audience gets to read

(Obregon and Waisbord, 2012). Those dominant ideas, Obregon and Waisbord argue, represent the hegemonic position of the health system, and in terms of the hegemonic approach, serve to reproduce and maintain the status quo, i.e., to support the interests of the elite, which the medical community is part of.

### Cut-and-paste industry's press releases

From the perspective of public health, an even bigger problem with this process is that as Corbett and Mori (1999) note, along with the government and the medical community, the powerful forces of the dominant ideology also include insurance companies and private industries, and the relations between those forces are interdependent. Thus, the industries' interests are in many cases those governing the journalistic texts. As Burton and Rowell (2003) put it:

> Few doctors have heard of the world's leading medical public relations companies. Yet barely a day passes without most doctors or their patients being exposed to messages that have been carefully crafted by these public relations companies, aimed at boosting sales of their clients' drugs.

A similar conclusion was drawn by Nelkin (1995) who argued that while PR practitioners help journalists to trace and translate news, they also "sell" science by promoting some discoveries and withholding others.

Indeed, studies have indicated that health journalists tend to favor stories on new drugs and technologies, and that the vast majority of medical and science news originates in press releases delivered by PR firms (de Semir et al., 1998; Entwistle, 1995; Schwitzer, 1992). These short communications, which are sent directly to journalists, are often written by the pharmaceutical companies, funding bodies or institutions supporting the clinical research, and are designed to attract favorable media attention to newly published research results (Yavchitz et al., 2012) and/or new drugs or technologies. The question is, to what extent drug companies succeed in this goal. It was argued that they are likely not only to attract attention, but in fact to influence the way health news is designed and framed (Park and Reber, 2010). Indeed, Yavchitz, et al. (2012) demonstrated just how influential those press releases are. Nearly half of the press releases and abstracts of scientific articles that their study examined contained "a spin" and, more importantly, that "spin" in the press releases was associated with "the spin" in the article abstracts.

The tendency of journalists to copy press releases and pre-packaged materials without carefully examining them was dubbed "churnalism" (Jackson, 2008). This questionable practice has been broadly criticized (Freimuth et al., 1984; Nelkin, 1995; Wilkins, 1987). Yet, in the digital age, as journalists are increasingly expected to produce more science news in less time, the phenomenon of "copy and paste journalism" has become even more prominent (Bauer and Bucchi, 2007; Lewis et al., 2008; Weitkamp, 2014; Weitkamp and Eidsvaag, 2014).

### Relying on industry press releases to describe infectious diseases and vaccines: the case of the Gardasil vaccine

When it comes to press releases prepared by the drug industry, this heavy reliance poses a particularly worrisome problem in terms of public health (Berzis, 2002). It is especially worrisome when the issue in focus concerns infectious diseases and outbreaks. In order to examine the extent to which industry press releases on new vaccines developed to prevent infectious diseases influence the way health news are designed and framed, we conducted a case study, focusing on the HPV (Human Papillomavirus) Gardasil vaccine. Through a qualitative content analysis, we explored how the Israeli media covered the information about the vaccine, the virus (HPV), and the disease linked to HPV (cervical cancer), during the period in which Gardasil was promoted by MSD Pharmaceutical (a subsidiary of Merck and Co., the vaccine manufacturer), and compared the media articles dealing with the subject and the company's press releases.

We identified and analyzed 18 press releases delivered by the company and its PR representatives from October 7, 2005, to June 17, 2012 – during the period of time in which the company was promoting the vaccine in two continuous campaigns, first, in order to accelerate its approval by the Israeli Health Ministry, and later on to encourage government funding, through its inclusion in the national immunization program vaccine. We also identified and analyzed 27 articles dealing with the Gardasil vaccine, which were published in three national daily newspapers (*Maariv, Yedioth Aharonot*, and *Haaretz*) and on popular websites (NRG and Ynet – the internet websites of *Maariv* and *Yedioth Aharonot*, and Doctors – the leading medical portal in Israel) during this period.

Then, a comparative analysis was carried out between the press releases and the articles. The comparative analysis showed that the media adopted the dominant framing presented in the company's press releases regarding the disease and the vaccine, and had used the data and statistics presented in those press releases.

### Framing the disease

The comparative analysis revealed troubling similarities in the frames chosen to describe the HPV and cervical cancer in the company's press release and the articles that followed. Although it seems that the journalists did rely on other sources in addition to the company's press releases – in general, the descriptions of the disease and the virus in most of the articles were similar to those in the press releases.

The two dominant frames found in both the press releases and the articles were:

*The chances of contracting HPV are extremely high.* This frame was accompanied by statistical data: 50%–80% of the population might be infected.

We found that more than a third of the articles (11 out of 27) chose this same frame to describe the disease, and cited these statistics presented in the press releases, to stress the high infection rates. Although as noted in Chapter 4, in most cases, the infection clears spontaneously without progressing to cervical cancer (Goldstein et al., 2009; Hathaway, 2012; National Advisory Committee on Immunization, 2007; Schiffman and Kjaer, 2003), this important information was omitted in the press releases. However, most of the media articles which described the HPV high rates (8 out of 11) did mention this information. Only in three of them was the information missing.

*There is a global "epidemic" of cervical cancer.* This frame creates the impression that the prevalence of cervical cancer throughout the world is extremely high, leading also to alarming global mortality rates. However, it ignores the substantial difference that exist, as noted in Chapter 4, in morbidity and mortality rates between the western and developing countries. While in developing countries, the morbidity and mortality rates are indeed high (Jemal et al., 2010; Parkin, 2006; WHO, 2015), in the western world, cervical cancer is actually relatively rare, following the wide adoption of the "pap test" (Connell and Hunt, 2010; Lowy, 2011), and in Israel in particular it is extremely rare (Beller, 2009; Hachim and Peled-Raz, 2007).We found that a third of the articles (9 out of 27) chose this same frame to describe the disease, highlighting the global statistics, instead of the local ones.

### The vaccine is the perfect solution

Another dominant frame employed in the company's press releases for health journalists concerns the vaccine itself, arguing that it has "an extra-ordinary efficiency in preventing cervical cancer," or even "a 99% efficiency." This frame relates to the vaccine as a "cervical cancer vaccine," instead of an "HPV vaccine," and furthermore, creates the impression that the vaccine is almost 100% efficient in preventing cervical cancer, while in fact, its goal and performance are much more modest. According to the clinical studies conducted by Merck itself, the vaccine indeed had a close to 100% efficiency in preventing infections, but only those caused by four HPV types (out of almost 100 that exist): the types 16 and 18, which are linked to approximately 70% of cases of cervical cancers, and the types 6 and 11, which account for 90% of genital warts. However, as the FDA (2006) stresses, "Gardasil did *not* protect against HPV types that are not in the vaccine," which are responsible for the remaining 30% of cervical cancer cases. In addition, findings from clinical studies indicate that while the vaccine's efficiency in preventing infection and precancerous lesions from types 16 and 18 is indeed close to 100% in women who have not yet been exposed to those types – its efficacy in preventing them in women who have already been exposed was only 44%, and the success in preventing precancerous lesions caused by all HPV types is merely 17%.

This means that even the precancerous processes are not prevented in the entire population, but, rather, mainly in women who have not been exposed to HPV (Beller, 2009; FDA, 2006).

Nevertheless, we found that more than half of the articles – 16 out of 27 – related to Gardasil's efficacy, and like the press releases, framed the vaccine as almost 100% efficient, while ignoring the important information regarding all the limitations described.

In addition to parroting the frames presented in the company's press releases, we found that 15 out of the 27 articles identified included interviews with medical experts suggested in the press releases.

On the other hand, we found that, like the press releases, the media articles rarely mentioned side effects or risks, the conflicts of interests of the medical experts interviewed, or the balancing views of experts expressing reservations regarding the accelerated promotion of the vaccine.

In conclusion, the findings from this case study indicate that although the media's adoption of the framing presented in the press releases is not absolute, and that in addition to the press releases, the media did use many times other sources to describe the disease and the vaccine, including the medical literature and formal sources, interviews with doctors etc., the "fingerprint" of the press releases is indeed evident in the media's framing of the disease and the vaccine.

### *Turning uncertainty into certainty*

In Stocking and Holstein's article about scientific ignorance (Stocking and Holstein, 1993), they note a number of approaches used by the media to deal with uncertainty. One approach is to turn scientific uncertainty into scientific certainty (Fahnestock, 1993; Weiss and Singer, 1988). Stocking and Holstein argue that in articles on popular science, journalists take into account their readers' lack of professional knowledge, prompting them to simplify complicated subjects and turn them into certainties.

Another tendency is the place certain journalists give to so-called maverick scientific theories. This is another facet of journalists' attempt to meet the challenge of popularity. These journalists report sensational theories, even if they turn out to be false, in the hope of arousing interest among their readers.

Dearing (1995) examined three such theories: (1) a 1990 earthquake prediction; (2) an alternative theory about the cause of AIDS; and (3) cold fusion. A content analysis of 393 news articles in 26 U.S. newspapers and a mail survey of the journalists who wrote those articles suggest that scientific theories, which are believed to be credible only by a minority of scientists, may be lent credibility in mass media stories, although the journalists themselves may think that the maverick scientists lacked credibility. The result is that an area of research appears more controversial and uncertain than most scientists believe it to be.

A prominent example is climate change. Along with the trend of giving "marginal" or "conspiratorial" theories a journalistic podium, journalists tend not to take a stand on controversial issues but to present "both sides of the story" in the name of "objectivity." But aside from striving to achieve objectivity, journalists tend not to take substantial positions. Furthermore, Stocking and Holstein (1993, pp. 204–205) note that the industry used the media cynically for years in order to plant doubt while facts piled up against smoking, with various journalists publishing studies that were funded by the tobacco industry. The very quotation of "other" pro-smoking studies created the false impression that the smoking issue had two sides. Thus, the media contributed to confusing the public and delaying health-promoting behavior change.

In their book, *Merchants of Doubt*, about the way scientists obscured the truth on issues from tobacco smoking to global warming, Oreskes and Conway (2011, p. 9) argue that journalists have played an active role in the industry's duplicity, and ask rhetorically: "Why did the press continue to quote them, year after year, even as their claims were shown, one after another, to be false"? Oreskes and Conway raised doubts as to the media's ability to distinguish between a real study and a commercially-driven tendentious study. They argue that journalists' attempts to make their reports balanced helped the industry to introduce confusing and conflicting messages to the public.

Stocking charges that not only did the media serve as a pawn for the industry, but it also betrayed its mission by failing to expose the political and economic mechanisms that prevent or delay studies of certain issues. By not always acting to expose the context in which studies are conducted, namely, who stood behind the study and what their interests were, the media contributed to strengthening and deepening "ignorance claims."

Notwithstanding the journalistic ethics (IFJ, 1986), which require accuracy, fairness, and public accountability in the reporting of credible information and its transmission to the public, still, as the Gardasil case study illustrates, journalists often serve as agents of the authorities and industry.

Another example is the alarming way the Dutch media chose to cover the 2009 influenza A (H1N1) pandemic (Vasterman and Ruigrok, 2013). Likewise, in the study we conducted during the 2009 H1N1 crisis, analyzing the transcripts of press conferences held by the WHO and the CDC during the outbreak, we found that the journalists' initial tendency was to promote the "epidemic" without a serious investigation of the element of uncertainty (which we discuss in detail below).

There are number of reasons for the journalists' heavy reliance on experts – both officials and experts with ties to the industry, and the failure of many reporters to address the various stakeholders in the risk communication circle. Largely, these problems stem from the complexity that characterizes health issues, their technical nature and the special expertise required to understand them. In many aspects, health journalists' work is similar to that of scientists.

According to Miranda, Vercellesi, and Bruno, just like any scientist, a good journalist

> should know how to find the latest information (the sources), how to assess it (the quality and authoritativeness), how to analyze and filter it (selection), how to deal with too many sources of information, sometimes case biased by conflicting interests (balance). The journalist must, in addition, know how to translate it to render it accessible and useful to the general public (dissemination), and how to use it best.
>
> (2004, p. 267)

Yet, this ideal similarity is often impaired by the fact that many health journalists lack the technical background, knowledge, training, and skills necessary to report on advanced scientific topics, to interpret statistics and to fully assess sources (Hinnant and Len-Ríos, 2009; Levi, 2001; Miranda et al., 2004; Voss, 2002). These limitations, as well as the time and space constraints and the demand to shorten and simplify complicated health issues, contribute to distortions in their coverage (Finer et al., 1997; Levi, 2001; Nelkin, 1996) and increase their tendency to rely on official and industry experts without delving into their motives and interests. Often, journalists are unaware of the powerful forces operating behind the marketing of a vaccine or medication. In addition, some of them have close ties or even friendships with representatives of the industry or the authorities, which may lead to biased reporting.

Yet, journalists not only fail to disclose the conflicting interests of various stakeholders, but are not always transparent about their own conflicting interests. As Stocking argued:

> If journalists tend to not reveal the constructed nature of ignorance claims and the interests they serve, they are even less likely to reveal their own interests with respect to the use of ignorance claims: their individual interests in protecting the environment or the economy, for example, or their organization's economic interests.
>
> (Stocking and Holstein, 1993, p. 205)

The absence of a discussion in the media about the stakeholders behind health coverage led Schwartz and colleagues to publish an article entitled "Who's watching the watchdogs?" (Schwartz et al., 2008). The article aimed to promote awareness and provoke debate about the education of journalists by industry, the press awards given by industry, and the conflicts of interest involved in the practice of journalism. Moreover, critics of science journalists have emphasized that they should disclose whether industry companies have paid for a journalist's travel expenses or for other gifts (Thacker, 2015).

Investigative journalism is supposed to reveal ulterior motives versus facts and fight what Zuckerman (2003) terms "checkbook" science (research undertaken to support marketing claims).

### Detached watchdog or opportunist facilitator? Virtual press meetings in the 2009 H1N1 outbreak

The seminal investigation by Bob Woodward and Carl Bernstein, which uncovered the illegal activities in the Watergate scandal that led to President Nixon's resignation in 1974, gave rise to the metaphor of journalists as watchdogs. This is a positive metaphor that portrays the role of journalists as vital, and as an expression of the soul of democracy.

In this era of changing media climate, along with powerful economic forces and religious and cultural wars, the question is how that metaphor is holding up. How do the power relations, which Bourdieu claimed range between autonomy and heteronomy, play out in the world of journalism, and specifically in health reporting (Benson, 2005)?

Over the years, researchers have tried to characterize the journalists' role in terms of level of journalistic interventionism (Hanitzsch, 2007). The scale ranges from the perception of the journalist as uninvolved/objective in public life (economic, political, health) at one end, to involved/influential at the other end (Deuze, 2005; Donsbach, 2008; Donsbach and Patterson, 2004).

A world-wide survey of 1800 journalists in 18 countries by Hanitzsch (2011) provided four journalistic profiles: (1) the populist disseminator; (2) the detached watchdog; (3) the critical change agent; and (4) the opportunist facilitator. The aforesaid study actually refines the scale of journalistic interventionism with the detached watchdog at one end of the scale and the critical change agent, on the other. What they both have in common is that "they articulate their skeptical and critical attitudes towards the government and business elites" (Hanitzsch, 2011, p. 485).

The difference between these two types of journalists is that the detached watchdog (an iteration of the classical watchdog) decidedly avoids, advocating for social change, influencing public opinion, and setting the political agenda – unlike their colleagues. At the other end are the populist disseminator and the opportunist facilitator, who share a lack of criticism of the government's power mechanisms.

Our analysis of press conferences during the H1N1 2009 outbreak illustrates the role played by journalists. The purpose of this study, as we describe in detail in Chapter 4, was to examine the communication between two central health authorities – the World Health Organization (WHO) and the Centers for Disease Control and Prevention (CDC), and the media, during the 2009 outbreak of the H1N1 influenza virus. The virtual press briefings held by both organizations during the outbreak and published by them provided an opportunity to examine the media's response during the outbreak, the different issues that the journalists focused on and asked about, and the ways in which they related to important issues, such as the decision to declare the H1N1 as a pandemic, the decision to produce vaccines in an accelerated process, and transparency regarding possible conflicts of interest and the decision-making process. These press conferences addressed epidemiological issues, coordination and management, and risk communication.

We would like to discuss two salient issues in risk communication. The first is communicating a crisis as an epidemic. The second is communicating the efficacy of the vaccine. Regarding both of these issues, we argue that a bleak picture emerges: the journalists functioned as respondents rather than leaders of the conversation, revealing the impotence of those who were assigned by the public to be the watchdogs of public health.

### Concern about downplaying the disease

Despite their confusion and lack of clarity regarding the criteria and the issue of severity, the main issue the journalists investigated during the period until the WHO's declaration was what they viewed as *the delay in the declaration of the pandemic*. Even though they were rather confused about the severity and the spread of the disease, it seems that they were anxious for the WHO to declare a pandemic, and kept asking why the organization had not yet raised the level of alert and moved from Phase 5 to Phase 6. Moreover, the journalists were mainly concerned that the authorities were downplaying the disease. Few journalists expressed concerns that the declaration might be unnecessary or that the authorities might be moving to Phase 6 too fast.

The following quotes illustrate the impatience and the pressure exerted by the journalists on the WHO to declare a pandemic:

> I wish if you could address the question of *why there seems to be so much reluctance on going to Phase 6*. It is a very clear definition ... What is to be lost by saying that it is spreading in the community in more than one place – which it obviously is – more than one region, *we are going to go to Phase 6 and it is a mild Phase 6. Why not just bite the bullet?*
>
> (WHO, 2009b, p. 3)

> Regarding the WHO announcement, there was speculation or even expectation that it might happen for weeks and weeks and weeks. *Now that it's finally happened, was that delay in some way beneficial in terms of the public understanding that it wasn't as severe as it might have been at the beginning?* Can you comment on that?
>
> (CDC, 2009)

> I wanted to follow up on David Brown's question. He asked, I thought sensibly, *why not bite the bullet and raise it to level 6 if it meets level 6?* The response was: what is the gain, this could be the panic, this could be the cynicism, but isn't that the other danger that if WHO changes its rules in the middle of the game, and appears to bend with the political pressure, that you create cynicism as well? *If it looks like WHO will bend with the political pressure, then it might do it with another public health*

*crisis and there is a loss of confidence in WHO.* There are other times when this question has been raised, for instance, when there might have been room for criticism with China during its silence in the early days of the SARS crisis, there might be criticism now with Indonesia for withholding viral samples. Isn't it important for WHO to maintain its credibility by sticking to its rules when it sets them?

(WHO, 2009b, p. 5)

The third period analyzed in this study relates to the press conference held on August 10, 2010, in which the WHO's senior officials declared the end of Phase 6. In contrast to the earlier press conferences held during periods I and II, this conference, in which the end of Phase 6 was announced, was characterized by blatant journalistic criticism and skepticism. It is as though the declaration awakened the media, and while earlier they served more as the WHO's mouthpiece than as the public watchdog – when the outbreak was over, they finally started to reclaim this role. The following question shows that there was a year-long delay before the journalists' criticism of the decision to declare a pandemic. "I just wanted to ask Dr Chan, are you still convinced that you made the right call in June of 2009 to declare the pandemic, *in view of the heavy criticism that followed?*" (WHO, 2010, p. 2).

The above quote also illustrates the fact that instead of initiating the criticism of and the inquiry into the WHO's conduct during the H1N1 outbreak and leading it, the journalists actually trailed behind the public criticism after it was voiced, and even this follow-up was too late – when the outbreak was already over. Another example indicates the problem of the accusations raised against the WHO of hyping the pandemic: "*The WHO was accused of hyping the pandemic* and I'm wondering whether this might pose problems for you in the future if and when a new pandemic arises?" (WHO, 2010, p. 7).

It is also worth noting the passive verb form the journalists used when they directed criticism towards the WHO – "the WHO *was accused* of hyping the pandemic"; "the heavy criticism *that followed.*" This use of the verb form gives the impression that even at this point, the journalists wanted to distance themselves from the criticism being voiced.

The declaration of the end of the pandemic also served as a wake-up call for the journalists to start asking why the WHO took so long to downgrade the pandemic – a question that in turn raises the question of why the media took so long to ask: "*Several countries started scaling back their H1N1 efforts some months ago, yet WHO held back on downgrading the pandemic phase until now. Why did they take so long?*" (WHO, 2010, p. 3).

The journalists also wanted to know if there were lessons learned from the year of the outbreak, and whether those lessons and experiences would change the response to pandemics in the future: "Dr. Chan, given the experience and evidence you've gathered over the last year, *will you change anything in the guidelines to respond to a new pandemic* that might break out in the future?" (WHO, 2010, p. 7).

### When will the vaccine be approved? And, wait, is it even safe?

Since, according to the WHO officials, the spread of the disease, and not its severity, was the central criterion in declaring the disease – a question the journalists should have raised was why it was so urgent to introduce a vaccine. In the first period, it seems that they were actually interested in *speeding up the development and the production of the vaccine.*

> I understand that the vaccine has some seed stocks to pile up and then full-scale manufacturing. *Is there a day, a week in time that WHO has set to make the decision whether to go to full-scale manufacturing?*
>
> (WHO, 2009a, p. 4)

In the second period, in contrast to the theme of speeding up the vaccine production, the second theme related to the new vaccines at this stage relates to vaccine safety. The following quotes demonstrate that at this stage, the journalists started to ask significant questions about safety issues, such as side effects and risks:

> I wonder with the accelerated safety tests that will be necessary, how many subjects will you expect to have tested and *how can experts draw conclusions about safety from these tests, when the vaccine has been put into hundreds of millions of people?*
>
> (WHO, 2009c, p. 5)

> Could I ask you to just repeat very briefly the European regulations and *how the Europeans are going to be testing the new vaccines?*
>
> (WHO, 2009d, p. 5)

In the final period, the journalists finally dared to ask for transparency regarding the money that the WHO had received during the outbreak. But even at this point only one single question was raised, and this was not followed by more critical questions, such as who exactly donated the money and how much was received from each pharmaceutical company involved: "Do you know how much money WHO received specifically to deal with H1N1 over the past year and what it was spent on?" (WHO, 2010, p. 3).

Glaringly absent from those press conferences was effective risk communication discourse. Critical questions attempting to expose the mechanisms and conflicts of interest between the WHO and the industry were rarely asked, nor was there an effective discussion of the WHO decision-making process and of disparities found between the declaration of an epidemic and reality. Criticism voiced by journalists towards the end of the meetings about the WHO decision-making was ineffective for two reasons. One, as we argued, is that the criticism was voiced by the journalists only after having been raised by the general public on the social networks, so that the journalists did not spearhead the exposure but rather trailed behind the public. Second, as we mentioned, the journalists petitioned for the declaration of an epidemic and marketing of the vaccine and that is why the criticism they leveled later appeared ineffective, slanted by political correctness, and even artificial. Instead of serving as watchdogs, the journalists emerged as opportunist facilitators. They were most likely to support official policies and convey a positive image of the health, and of the political and pharmaceutical representatives. Despite characteristics of uncertainty in the epidemic emergence and despite questions of effectiveness and safety, the press created a false appearance of "certainty." The search for sensation (epidemic mongering) and the tendency to hype the instant publication of a new discovery led health reporters to tend to resort to pre-scripted materials from official sources, which, to use a term from Stocking, contributed to "strengthening ignorance claims," as far as the public was concerned.

### New media and the "good ol' press"

The technological revolution of new media raises one of the most important questions for the press: has the Internet strengthened the press as democracy's watchdog, weakened it, or made no significant difference? The Internet revolution generated far-reaching changes in the public sphere. Manovich called it, "the shift of all of our culture to computer-mediated forms of production, distribution and communication" (2001, p. 43).

New media have increased interactivity and have made it possible for people to share and voice their opinions everywhere and at any time (Vogt, 2011, p. 17). The boundless Internet space has led to the "death of distance" (Cairncross, 2001), not only by reducing geographic space but mainly by canceling social distance. The Internet has provided a tailwind for globalization, in which citizens from all over the world can create (mainly on the social media and creative platforms), express their opinions, and respond to press reports appearing online all over the world.

Manovich has argued that the Internet revolution created a new individualism in the 21st-century mass media. "Every citizen can construct her own custom lifestyle and 'select' her ideology from a large number of choices. Rather than pushing the same objects to a mass audience, marketing now tries to target each individual separately" (Manovich, 2001, p. 60).

The different New Media platforms gave rise to new communication methods in the mass media, especially in relation to the interaction between people in the public global sphere.

Vin Crosbie (2002) has demonstrated three different kinds of communication media. He pinpointed interpersonal media as "one to one," mass media as "one to many," and finally New Media as individuation media or "many to many." He argued that:

> The millions of computers interconnected through the Internet can acquire, sort, package, and transmit information in as many ways as there

are individual people. They can establish those communications simultaneously. And they allow each participant (senders and receivers) to share equal simultaneous control.

(Crosbie, 2002, p. 6)

The Internet Revolution has proven to be a challenge for the print media: into the realm of traditional media new market forces have entered, which led to the closure of newspapers, worker layoffs, imposed pay cuts (Mahmud, 2009; Yap, 2009), slashed the size of physical newspapers, and forced the transition of media outlets to web-only publication (Kirchhoff, 2009).

Whereas in the traditional media the writers were journalists with professional identities, the New Media blurred those boundaries beyond recognition and created the concept of citizen journalism (Bowman and Willis, 2003) – citizens who write on social media, express their opinions and become information arbiters and opinion leaders for their friends and acquaintances. The Internet environment blurred the boundaries between the "consumer" and the "informator" (Creeber and Martin, 2009). Now professional journalists actually must compete with the citizen who in the past played the passive role of reader and now has become a responder or even an information generator.

In the New Media, citizens are empowered (Bennett, 2003) to report on their political experiences while being held to high standards of information quality and community values. Journalists used to working in the traditional media under time and space constraints have had to change their work patterns beyond recognition.

The speed of information transmission allows journalists to obtain information without leaving the room (Quinn, 2002). Diverse materials and information sources, including reactions from different publics that are hard to access, can now be obtained with a keyboard stroke. However, this speed sometimes creates problematic situations where journalists are forced to publish before checking their sources. This abundance of information can also lead to "copy and paste journalism" (Gunter, 2003).

McNair argues that the proliferation of news platforms has led to a transition from elite journalism to "multiple publics, connected in key ways" (2009, p. 213). Online journalism offers its audiences a more multidimensional view than old, traditional journalism. In addition, multimedia formats also allow news to be presented in innovative and interesting ways (Kenix, 2013).

The question is whether the transition to the Internet's conditions of time and space, which has improved access to stories and sources, has also improved journalists' professionalism. In other words, does multiplicity always translate into polycentrality and diversity? Quandt (2008) argues to the contrary, that the transition to new online platforms might have increased journalists' dependence on external sources of information, such as governmental representatives, due to the constant pressure of deadlines, which allows them little time to validate data.

To answer this question, we must conduct various empirical studies in the field of journalism and New Media. This research field is still in its infancy. However, we can already detect a trend that indicates that health reporters are following their old patterns in the New Media. The work of health journalists has particular characteristics, two of which we will discuss here. First, health journalists prefer official information sources and especially officials in government organizations (Altheide, 2006; Seletzky and Lehman-Wilzig, 2010). Second, health journalists give pride of place to science and therefore they tend to give space to doctors in their reports (Lariscy et al., 2010; Len-Ríos et al., 2009).

We conducted a study of the 2013 polio outbreak in Israel as a case study to examine the sources used in various online platforms, and tried to understand whether the New Media led to a new discourse on health-related topics, or simply reproduced the traditional discourse using new tools (Gesser-Edelsburg, Walter and Shir-Raz, 2016). We found that news websites were more likely to rely on Ministry of Health representatives than on Facebook, forums, and blogs. This finding suggests that despite using a new platform, health journalists working in mainstream media still operated in the same way as they did using traditional news platforms. This may be because the journalists themselves did not change their fundamental approach to writing on health issues. In other words, while the Internet has enabled journalists to make their writing more accessible, to distribute it more quickly and to a broader audience, it has not altered their approach to and use of external sources. Yet, these results also suggest that the Internet has gradually eroded the level of journalistic reporting in terms of the type and diversity of sources cited. Another plausible explanation that we raised in our discussion relates to the fact that health journalists (both those who write for newspapers and those who write for news websites) use their personal connections with government officials in order to receive exclusive information that the public cannot readily obtain. In this regard, the journalist-source relationship might represent a clash between different interests, as sources work to further their preferred interpretation of the events by capitalizing on the credibility usually associated with the traditional press. As for medical professionals, we found that news websites did not cite experts more than other platforms did. Ostensibly, this finding seems to contradict conclusions from studies on health journalists working in the traditional media, which concludes that they often cite medical professionals and academic centers as sources. Yet, these discrepancies can be explained by the nature of the situation. While, as noted above, journalists routinely tend to rely mainly on physicians, scientists, medical professionals and academic centers as sources – in crisis situations, their first inclination would be to turn first to decision-makers and official sources, rather than to medical professionals. Thus, we might speculate that during a potentially deadly outbreak, government officials are perceived as more accountable and better informed than medical professionals.

The tendency of health reporters to rely on official sources was also evident in other crises, such as the Ebola, SARS, etc. Compared to "ordinary" situations where journalists can turn to doctors and other sources, in crises characterized by time pressure, they rely mainly on government sources.

Despite the significant potential of New Media to facilitate access to access diverse sources and publics, and verify information sources, it is evident that journalists still prefer to use old and even populist methods. The studies that were conducted found that mainstream newspapers reproduce stories for their websites and actually create more of the same (Singer, 1997). Many health journalists continue to publish mainly press releases and marketing contents from the pharmaceutical companies and to serve as the mouthpieces of official sources during epidemic crises.

Furthermore, the discourse on the social networks is sometimes more poignant and challenging than the reports of many journalists. Instead of the competition created by the New Media challenging the journalists and leading them to use original and creative methods of communication that the non-professional blogger is unable to utilize, many journalists prefer to look for a good and populist story rather than exposing corruption and generating an in-depth discussion of issues in controversy in the scientific community. Paradoxically, as we showed, journalists, who served for years as the industry's mouthpieces for sowing doubt, such as in the case of the tobacco industry and global warming denial (Oreskes and Conway, 2011), tend to avoid exposing issues that really do contain scientific uncertainty and usually prefer to communicate the official political stance of the health organizations. The absence of an in-depth discussion in the media and the weakening power of journalism to serve as the public watchdog undermine democracy's ability to maintain an interactive public sphere that works in favor of public health.

### *A journalism jail*

Yet, the responsibility for the media's weakening ability to serve as the watchdogs of public health cannot entirely be placed at the feet of the journalists. In a report published in 2014 entitled, "Ebola and Freedom of Expression in West Africa," the Media Foundation for West Africa (MFWA) pointed to an "upsurge in general intolerance towards the media in the affected countries, including attacks on and arrests and detentions of journalists, closures of media houses and increased levels of official and unofficial censorship among the media" (Hagan, 2014; MFWA, 2014).

Although physical attacks and arrests or detentions of journalists are rare in western countries, the value of free media might nevertheless be compromised when doctors and organizations paid by the pharmaceutical industry are trying to censor vaccine information, and when journalists who do "dare" to stand guard as watchdogs are slandered and smeared by those experts. At the annual meeting in 2014 of the Association for Health Care Journalists, Dr. Paul Offit, the chief of infectious disease at Children's Hospital of Philadelphia, stated that there should be a "journalism jail" for reporters who write stories about risks involved with vaccines and people who die following vaccination (Kroll, 2014). Six years earlier, in 2008, Sharil Attkisson, a former CBS News investigative correspondent, revealed in a CBS *Evening News* report, that Dr. Offit, one of the most widely-quoted defenders of vaccine safety, who stated that babies can tolerate "10,000 vaccines at once," has strong industry ties. According to Attkisson's investigative news report, entitled "How Independent Are Vaccine Defenders?," Offit holds a $1.5 million research chair at Children's Hospital, funded by Merck, the vaccine manufacturer. He also holds a patent on an anti-diarrhoea vaccine, Rotateq, for which he has received unspecified royalties (estimated to be in the millions of dollars) (Attkisson, 2008). In response, Offit smeared Attkisson, arguing that she "lied" when she noted in her report that he failed to inform CBS about exactly how much money he and his Children's Hospital of Philadelphia were paid by Merck, and that CBS News sent a "mean spirited and vituperative" email "over the signature of Sharyl Attkisson" stating "You're clearly hiding something." He made these defamatory accusations in an interview to the *OC Register*, a newspaper in Orange County. Yet, in 2011, the newspaper published a retraction, when documents provided by CBS News indicated Offit did not disclose his financial relationships with Merck (*OC Register*, 2011). The importance of a free media, able to protect public interest is guaranteed under the International Covenant on Economic, Social and Cultural Rights (ICESCR). Restricting information about infectious diseases, outbreaks, and vaccines by hampering freedom of expression could be harmful to the public.

## Part 2: The role of medical experts

Scientists and doctors often criticize journalists for distorting medical information, for favoring sensations and for "panic-mongering" (Hargreaves, 2001). Indeed, as noted above, scholars have often pointed out the differences between these two professionals. For example, while journalists favor sensations and tend to use anecdotal or rhetorical evidence, doctors and scientists work to inform and educate the public and stress the importance of disease prevention. They rely on evidence and proceed by careful peer-reviewed trial and error (Berzis, 2002; Hargreaves, 2001; Leask et al., 2010; Nelkin, 1996). Yet, as numerous examples presented in this book illustrate, not infrequently, doctors and scientists themselves are the ones accounting for the bias, distortions and exaggerations in the media. As Sumner et al. (2014) has demonstrated, misleading health-related news is often the result of exaggerated and inaccurate press releases, written by scientists in academic institutions.

Health organizations and health authorities view health professionals as representatives of the establishment, whose role is to mediate between the organization and the public. Furthermore, according to official ECDC documents, health professionals constitute "the message" and the voice of the organization: "Target health professionals, not only to pass the message, but also 'to be' the message" (ECDC, 2012, p. 30).

The perception of doctors as "the voice" of health organizations is rooted in the "Third party technique" – a strategy widely employed by the industry. Instead of using a company representative (who would have low credibility) as spokesperson, this strategy is based on recruiting an apparently independent messenger (whose credibility would be perceived as higher in the eyes of the target audience) to present the messages put forward by the company. In other words, the strategy helps corporations to separate the message from what could be seen as a self-interested messenger (Burton and Rowell, 2003). As Merrill Rose, executive vice president of the Porter/Novelli PR firm, has put it: "Put your words in someone else's mouth" (Rose, 1991). In the pharmaceutical field, this "someone else" are doctors and patients, medical associations and patient organizations, who are recruited, trained, funded and fostered by the drug companies, to promote their drugs and medical treatments (Burton and Rowell, 2003; Elliott, 2010; Goldacre, 2013; Rampton and Stauber, 2002).

As far as the companies are concerned, the idea of putting physicians at the forefront of the message is a very efficient strategy, which promises that their messages would be perceived as reliable and convincing. Not only are doctors considered experts and authority when it comes to diseases and drugs (Elliott, 2010), but in contrast to journalists, are at consistently the upper end of trustworthiness rankings (Hargreaves, 2001). Senior doctors and heads of medical associations, who are considered key opinion leaders, are particularly influential (Burton and Rowell, 2003). When those leading experts are interviewed in the media and recommend on a certain drug, treatment or vaccine, while serving as a third party for the industry, their recommendations has a substantial influence on the public (Gosden and Beder, 2001). Yet, the close relationship that exist between the pharma and physicians and medical associations has been criticized, since economic relations were found between these parties, which may lead to conflicts of interests (Brody and Light, 2011; De Ferrari et al., 2014; Komesaroff, 2010; Moynihan et al., 2013; Norris et al., 2004; Rothman, et al., 2009).

Health organizations and health ministries employed physicians as the messengers, requiring public health professionals not only to mediate between the organizations' directives and the public, but also to market vaccinations. In this case, the strategy does not exactly come under the definition of "Third party technique," as for the organizations, the physicians are not "someone else," but rather, a part of the health system. Nevertheless, recruiting doctors is no less vital to these organizations than to the industry, since by the very fact they are governmental and/or political organizations, the public trusts them less than physicians (Hargreaves, 2001).

### Are healthcare workers part of the system or part of the public?

Healthcare workers have been the subject of many studies as they are uniquely positioned as an extension of the healthcare system, while also being a part of the public, therefore comprising a risk group. The fact that healthcare workers belong to the general public is evident from the findings of studies in the scientific literature that examined the general public's barriers compared with those of healthcare professionals in relation to vaccinations. These findings contrast with claims in risk communication literature that cast healthcare workers as "experts" who process information about risk differently from the public. The "mental models" approach (Morgan et al., 2002) indicates a differentiation between experts and the public, concluding that studies need to be conducted with the public in order to shape risk communication messages to address the gaps in the audience's knowledge.

However, even though healthcare workers are a "professional" public, it was found that similar to the general public, they are often reluctant to vaccinate, and their barriers are similar as well, including concerns about side effects, the novelty of the vaccination, and lack of faith in its efficacy and in the severity of the disease (Smedley et al., 2007; Weingarten et al., 1989; Willis and Wortley, 2007). Studies indicate that both healthcare workers who choose to vaccinate (Hakim et al., 2011; Rebmann et al., 2012a, 2012b) and those who do not encode the same epidemiological data in different ways (Piccirillo and Gaeta, 2006; Wicker et al., 2010).

### Cognitive dissonance

Healthcare professionals' decision to vaccinate depends on their faith in the health system and its message. When an organization promotes a vaccine and the healthcare professional trusts the vaccine and trusts the organization, there is no controversy. The problems begin when there is a discrepancy between different factors in the equation.

Healthcare professionals often experience cognitive dissonance (Festinger, 1985), wherein their professional obligation to recommend vaccination clashes with their personal values and perceptions. The literature rarely deals with the processes underlying this ambivalence and the barriers and concerns that challenge or undermine their professional attitudes. This dissonance is often reflected in the gap that exists between the declarative level – in which healthcare workers recommend that their patients vaccinate, and the behavioral level – their reluctance to vaccinate with the very same vaccines they have recommended. A prominent example is the seasonal flu vaccine. Although they recommend that patients vaccinate each winter, only a small percentage of healthcare workers get vaccinated themselves (Aguilar-Díaz et al., 2011; Chittaro et al., 2009; Seale et al., 2010; Takayanagi et al., 2007; Vírseda et al., 2010; Wicker et al., 2009). For example, the Centers for Disease Control and Prevention estimated that only 62% of healthcare professionals received the seasonal flu vaccine in the 2009–2010 season (CDC, 2010), and in the 2010–2011 season, 63.5% of HCP reported influenza vaccination (CDC, 2011).

The "solution" to reducing the gap between declarations and actual behavior, often heard on the organizational level, is to "crack down," by obliging healthcare workers to get vaccinated. The obligation can be in the form of legislation or alternatively, through punishments on the systemic level. Yet, turning a voluntary act into a mandatory one raises obvious ethical and legal issues (Anikeeva et al., 2009; Eidelman and Karni, 2014; Israel Medical Association Legal Department, 2014). Nevertheless, the idea of obliging medical personnel to vaccinate often resurfaces in internal discussions in government ministries, or is reflected by the exercise of authority or force by governmental bodies that push hospital directors to pressure their staff. For example, in 2009, the State of New York issued a seasonal and pandemic influenza vaccination mandate for healthcare workers (Daines, 2009). In Israel, the management of several hospitals decided in 2014 to "mark" doctors and nurses who received flu vaccinations, by requiring them to carry tags which indicated they had been vaccinated (Eidelman and Karni, 2014). In October 2015, the Israeli Health Ministry instructed hospitals and HMOs' managements to require that all medical personnel be vaccinated against influenza (Doctors Only Staff, 2015).

### *Gap between guidelines at the international level and their implementation at the local level*

Healthcare workers play a key role in supporting the public during an epidemic outbreak, especially primary care providers (Lam and McGeer, 2011), by mediating guidelines to the public and adapting the message to their needs. In the WHO guidelines and reports regarding the 2009 H1N1 outbreak, the instructions for healthcare workers were mainly procedural. While they received instructions regarding whom to vaccinate, when, and how, they did not receive instructions on how to contend with fears, questions, and skepticism.

In a study we conducted in Israel during the 2009 H1N1 outbreak (Gesser-Edelsburg et al., 2014a), to examine how the guidelines were implemented at the local level, we found that while most of the healthcare workers were familiar with the guidelines regarding whom and how to vaccinate, they stated that they received no guidance on how to discuss the vaccination. Nurses said that the general impression was that the public should be forced to get vaccinated and that this process lacked active explanation: "We had written protocols ... what we needed to know, who would get it ... " (a senior nurse). "We were instructed to vaccinate and that's it" (a nurse); "There were just general guidelines" (a senior nurse) (Gesser-Edelsburget al., 2014a, p. 163).

Another aspect of uncertainty that emerges from the reports (2009–2011) refers to the vaccine itself. Many questions were raised regarding its safety and its capacity to prevent infection, issues which inhibited vaccination compliance. Other uncertainties related to the vaccine included availability, safety, efficacy and priority group distribution (Brennan and Hall, 2009). The WHO and CDC reported: "The emergence of a novel pandemic H1N1 (pH1N1) influenza strain presented many communication challenges for public health officials. There were 'unknowns' about the disease, such as severity and spread during the initial stages" (Brennan and Hall, 2009; Lam and McGeer, 2011). Among healthcare workers, our research exposed two tendencies. The first consisted of healthcare workers who followed the pandemic and vaccine guidelines without being troubled by uncertainty. The second consisted of healthcare workers who followed the WHO and CDC guidelines ambivalently, feeling many questions had been left unanswered:

> On the one hand, we received guidelines to vaccinate, but we still had questions about this process ... there were many unknowns ... how could I vaccinate someone and convince him when I myself had doubts? (nurse).
>
> (Gesser-Edelsburg et al., 2014a, p. 164)

Furthermore, the healthcare workers said that although the epidemic was moderate in scale, communicating the vaccine was the only alternative they were given. "No alternative was presented" (a medic). "The vaccine was the only relevant solution at that time" (policy-maker) (Gesser-Edelsburg et al., 2014a, p. 164).

Further, it was found that although the guidelines of the WHO and CDC addressed conceptual elements such as communicating uncertainty, segmentation, and empowerment (of diverse stakeholders), there was a gap in implementation, according to our analysis of the findings in the empirical study.

In other words, there are WHO guidelines about the importance of transparency and inclusion, but, at the implementation level, healthcare workers find it difficult to mediate between the organizations and the establishment, on the one hand, and the public, on the other. This is because, like the public, they feel their questions are left unanswered and feel they are not sufficiently included in the process.

### Motivation not knowledge as a function of emotional involvement

The literature naturally tends to perceive healthcare workers as more knowledgeable than the general public about health issues. But the perception of healthcare workers as "experts" does not take into account data such as the different expertise of different healthcare workers; exposure to information sources (aside from the official health ministry guidelines); the motivation of the healthcare worker; their emotional involvement; and risk perception. All of the above influence their motivation to acquire knowledge, as well as their level of knowledge.

Two studies we conducted reveal that health professionals and the public have similar risk perceptions and knowledge about epidemics in an as-yet uninfected country. The studies were conducted in the context of two epidemics that received wide media coverage although not a single case was reported in Israel. The first examines the correlation between worry level and risk perception. It focuses on the emergence of Avian Influenza A (H7N9) in China in 2013, and illustrates the importance of healthcare professionals as a medium between health agencies and the public (Gesser-Edelsburg et al., 2014b). This study examined Israeli healthcare professionals' risk perceptions considering their unique positioning as representing the healthcare system while also part of the public, hence a risk group. We distributed an online survey using *Google Docs* to Israeli healthcare professionals and the general public in Israel. We found that when risk perception is relatively low, health-care professionals tend to base their attitudes toward vaccines on analytical knowledge ($Rc$ = .315, $p$<.05), whereas in situations with high risk perception, the results did not indicate any significant difference between Israeli health professionals and the Israeli general public: both groups based their attitudes more on emotions and personal experience than analytical knowledge.

The second example compares the level of knowledge of health care workers with that of the public concerning the Ebola virus, with reference to their sources of knowledge. The purpose of our study (Gesser-Edelsburg et al., 2015) was to examine what the Israeli public knew about Ebola. Using an online survey (n = 327), we analyzed the knowledge of healthcare workers compared to non-healthcare workers and each group's concerns about contracting the disease. In addition, we assessed the association between knowledge about Ebola versus concerns about contracting the disease. The main finding indicates that the Israeli public had knowledge about it ($M$ = 4.18, $SD$ = 0.83), despite the fact that the disease had not spread to Israel. No statistically significant difference was found between healthcare workers and non-healthcare workers in the knowledge score. Additionally, no statistically significant correlation was found between knowledge and worry levels. This finding undermines the assumption of the "mental model," that healthcare professionals have greater access to scientific information and are more likely to understand it (Gesser-Edelsburg, et al., 2015). We can interpret it in light of the fact that healthcare workers, like the general public, are exposed to information mainly via the media. Since Ebola did not occur in Israel, it is possible that the community of healthcare workers, doctors and nurses had been exposed to little if any professional discussions to which the general public had not been exposed. In addition, this study revealed that we must take into account that healthcare professionals do not necessarily have the comprehensive knowledge of virus experts. This group is often viewed as "expert," whereas it is actually a sub-group of the general public.

In light of the above, it appears that the organizations should change their attitudes towards healthcare workers. Healthcare workers are part of the general public. In order for them to serve as mediators between the organizations and the public, the organizations must recognize their concerns and fears, and include them in the process rather than merely giving them "guidelines" or "messages." Healthcare workers can be included in numerous ways, including setting up an online system where healthcare workers are free to voice their concerns and reservations.

Furthermore, the assumption that healthcare workers have access to "science" and therefore read more scientific literature than the general public must be critically revisited. As we indicate in our research, that assumption was refuted and requires further study. Therefore, healthcare workers should be encouraged to read scientific literature by sending them scientific studies and initiating discussions about them, also including studies that question the consensus. This would turn healthcare workers into an informed audience and partners in the process.

# References

Abramson, J. (2008). *Overdosed America: The Broken Promise of American Medicine.* New York: Harper Perennial.

Aguilar-Díaz, F. d. C., Jiménez-Corona, M. E., and Ponce-de-León-Rosales, S. (2011). Influenza vaccine and healthcare workers. *Archives of Medical Research*, 42(8), 652–657.

Allen, N., and Alexander, H. (2014). Ebola outbreak: America's first Ebola victim dies. *The Telegraph.* October 8. Available at: www.telegraph.co.uk/news/worldnews/ebola/11149331/Americas-first-Ebola-victim-Thomas-Eric-Duncan-dies-in-Dallas.html

Altheide, D. L. (2006). Terrorism and the politics of fear. *Cultural Studies ↔ Critical Methodologies*, 6(4), 415–439.

Anikeeva, O., Braunack-Mayer, A., and Rogers, W. (2009). Requiring influenza vaccination for health care workers. *American Journal of Public Health*, 99(1), 24–29.

Attkisson, S. (2008). How independent are vaccine defenders? *CBS NEWS.* July 25, Available at: www.cbsnews.com/news/how-independent-are-vaccine-defenders/

Bakhtin, M. M. (1981). *The Dialogic Imagination: Four Essays* (trans. C. Ernerson and M. Holquist). Austin: University of Texas Press.

Bauer, M. W., and Bucchi, M. (2007). *Journalism, Science, and Society: Science Communication between News and Public Relations.* New York: Routledge.

Beller, U. (2009). The vaccine against cervical cancer: Truths, hope, and illusions. Available at: http://themedical.co.il/Article.aspx?f=12ands=2andid=2968 (accessed May 13, 2016).

Bennett, W. L. (2003). New media power: The internet and global activism. In N. Couldry and J. Curran (Eds.), *Contesting Media Power: Alternative Media Power in a Networked World* (pp. 17–38). Lanham, MD: Rowman and Littlefield.

Benson, R. (2005). Mapping field variation: Journalism in France and the United States. In R. Benson and E. Neveu (Eds.), *Bourdieu and the Journalistic Field* (pp. 85–112). Cambridge: Polity Press.

Berzis, M. (2002). Who will be responsible for the health of the media? *Harefuah*, 1(6), 44–46.

Bomlitz, L. J., and Brezis, M. (2008). Misrepresentation of health risks by mass media. *Journal of Public Health*, 30(2), 202–204.

Bowman, S., and Willis, C. (2003). *We Media: How Audiences Are Shaping the Future of News and Information.* Reston, VA: The Media Center at The American Press Institute.

Boyd, E. A., and Bero, L. A. (2000). Assessing faculty financial relationships with industry: A case study. *JAMA*, 284(17), 2209–2214.

Boyd, E. A., Cho, M. K., and Bero, L. A. (2003). Financial conflict-of-interest policies in clinical research: Issues for clinical investigators. *Academic Medicine*, 78(8), 769–774.

Brennan, B., and Hall, W. (2009). Putting Planning into Practice: The Communications Response to H1N1. A Global Communications conference sponsored by the Pan American Health Organization and the United States Department of Health and Human Services. Conference report and conclusions: Pan American Health Organization, Department of Health and Human Services USA, Washington, DC,22 July. Available at: www1.paho.org/cdmedia/riskcommguide/Putting%20Planning%20into%20Practice_GlobalComm_FinalReport_Eng.pdf

Brody, H., and Light, D. W. (2011). The inverse benefit law: How drug marketing undermines patient safety and public health. *American Journal of Public Health*, 101(3), 399–404.

Bubela, T. M., and Caulfield, T. A. (2004). Do the print media "hype" genetic research? A comparison of newspaper stories and peer-reviewed research papers. *Canadian Medical Association Journal*, 170(9), 1399–1407.

Burton, B., and Rowell, A. (2003). Unhealthy spin. *BMJ*, 326(7400), 1205–1207.

Cairncross, F. (2001). *The Death of Distance: How the Communications Revolution Is Changing our Lives*. Boston: Harvard Business School Press.

Caulfield, T. (2004). The commercialisation of medical and scientific reporting. *PLoS Medicine*, 1(3), e38.

CDC. (2009). Press briefing transcripts: CDC press conference on investigation of human cases of novel influenza A H1N1. June 11. Atlanta, GA: Centers for Disease Control and Prevention.

CDC. (2010). Interim results: Influenza A (H1N1) 2009 monovalent and seasonal influenza vaccination coverage among health-care personnel – United States, August 2009–January 2010. *Morbidity and Mortality Weekly Report*, 59(12), 357–362.

CDC. (2011). Influenza vaccination coverage among health-care personnel – United States, 2010–2011 influenza season. *Morbidity and Mortality Weekly Report*, 60(32), 1073–1077. Chittaro, M., Turello, D., Calligaris, L., et al. (2009). Impact of vaccinating HCWs on the ward and possible influence of avian flu threat. *Infection*, 37(1), 29–33.

Cole, B. J. (1975). Trends in science and conflict coverage in four metropolitan newspapers. *Journalism and Mass Communication Quarterly*, 52(3), 465–471.

Connell, E., and Hunt, A. (2010). The HPV vaccination campaign: A project of moral regulation in an era of biopolitics. *Canadian Journal of Sociology*, 35(1), 63–82.

Cook, D. M., Boyd, E. A., Grossmann, C., and Bero, L. A. (2007). Reporting science and conflicts of interest in the lay press. *PLoS ONE*, 2(12), e1266.

Corbett, J. B., and Mori, M. (1999). Medicine, media, and celebrities: News coverage of breast cancer, 1960–1995. *Journalism and Mass Communication Quarterly*, 76(2), 229–249.

Creeber, G., and Martin, R. (2009). *Digital Cultures: Understanding New Media*. Maidenhead: Open University Press.

Crosbie, V. (2002). What is new media? Available at: www.sociology.org.uk/as4mm3a.doc (accessed May 13, 2016).

Cunningham, R. M., and Boom, J. A. (2013). Telling stories of vaccine-preventable diseases: Why it works. *South Dakota Journal of Medicine*, Spec no: 21–26.

Daines, R. F. (2009). Mandatory flu vaccine for health care workers. Commissioner tells health care workers: Mandatory flu vaccine is in the best interest of patients and workers. Albany, NY: New York State, Department of Health.

Dearing, J. W. (1995). Newspaper coverage of maverick science: Creating controversy through balancing. *Public Understanding of Science*, 4(4), 341–361.

De Ferrari, A., Gentille, C., Davalos, L., Huayanay, L., and Malaga, G. (2014). Attitudes and relationship between physicians and the pharmaceutical industry in a public general hospital in Lima, Peru. *PLoS ONE*, 9(6), e100114.

de Semir, V., Ribas, C., and Revuelta, G. (1998). Press releases of science journal articles and subsequent newspaper stories on the same topic. *JAMA*, 280(3), 294–295. Deuze, M. (2005). What is journalism? Professional identity and ideology of journalists reconsidered. *Journalism*, 6(4), 442–464.

Dew, K. (1999). Epidemics, panic and power: Representations of measles and measles vaccines. *Health*, 3(4), 379–398.

Dew, K. (2012). *The Cult and Science of Public Health: A Sociological Investigation.* New York: Berghahn Books.

Diem, S. J., Lantos, J. D., and Tulsky, J. A. (1996). Cardiopulmonary resuscitation on television – Miracles and misinformation. *New England Journal of Medicine*, 334(24), 1578–1582.

Doctors Only Staff. (2015). The Ministry of Health requires all medical personnel to get vaccinated against flu . *Doctors Only*, October 8. Available at: http://doctorsonly. co.il/2015/10/102286/

Donsbach, W. (2008). Journalists' role perception. In W. Donsbach (Ed.), *The International Encyclopedia of Communication*, Vol. 6 (pp. 2605–2610). Oxford: Wiley-Blackwell.

Donsbach, W., and Patterson, T. E. (2004). Political news journalists: Partisanship, professionalism, and political roles in five countries. In F. Esser and B. Pfetsch (Eds.), *Comparing Political Communication: Theories, Cases, and Challenges* (pp. 251–270). Cambridge: Cambridge University Press.

Drazen, J. M., and Koski, G. (2000). To protect those who serve. *New England Journal of Medicine*, 343(22), 1643–1645.

ECDC. (2012). *Communication on Immunisation – Building Trust*. April. Available at: http://ecdc.europa.eu/en/publications/Publications/TER-Immunisation-and-trust. pdf

Eidelman, L., and Karni, T. (2014). *Influenza Vaccines for Doctors*. Ramat Gan: Israel Medical Association, Ethics Board.

Elliott, C. (2010). *White Coat, Black Hat: Adventures on the Dark Side of Medicine.* Boston: Beacon Press.

Entwistle, V. (1995). Reporting research in medical journals and newspapers. *BMJ*, 310 (6984), 920–923.

Fahnestock, J. (1993). Accommodating science: the rhetorical life of scientific facts. In M. W. McRae (Ed.), *The Literature of Science: Perspectives on Popular Scientific Writing* (pp. 17–36). Athens: University of Georgia Press.

Fairclough, N. (1989). *Language and Power*. New York: Longman.

Fantz, A. (2014). Doctor's death marks second U.S. Ebola fatality . *CNN*. November 18. Available at: http://edition.cnn.com/2014/11/17/health/ebola-u-s-/

FDA. (2006). Gardasil (Human Papillomavirus Vaccine) questions and answers, June 8, 2006. Available at: www.fda.gov/BiologicsBloodVaccines/Vaccines/Questionsa boutVaccines/ucm096052.htm (accessed May 13, 2016).

Festinger, L. (1985). *A Theory of Cognitive Dissonance.* Stanford, CA: Stanford University Press.

Finer, D., Tomson, G., and Björkman, N. M. (1997) Ally, advocate, analyst, agenda-setter? Positions and perceptions of Swedish medical journalists. *Patient Education and Counseling*, 30(1), 71–81.

Fisher, J., Gandy, O. H., Jr., and Janus, N. Z. (1981). The role of popular media in defining sickness and health. In E. G. McAnany, J. Schnitman and N. Janus (Eds.), *Communication and Social Structure: Critical Studies in Mass Media Research* (pp. 240–257). New York: Praeger.

Freimuth, V. S., Greenberg, R. H., DeWitt, J., and Romano, R. M. (1984). Covering cancer: Newspapers and the public interest. *Journal of Communication*, 34(1), 62–73.

Friedman, P. J. (2002). The impact of conflict of interest on trust in science. *Science and Engineering Ethics*, 8(3), 413–420.

Gamson, W. A. (1992). *Talking Politics.* New York: Cambridge University Press.

Gans, H. J. (1979). *Deciding What's News: A Study of CBS Evening News, NBC Nightly News, Newsweek, and Time.* New York: Pantheon Books.

Gerbner, G. (1969). Dimensions of violence in television drama. A staff report to the National Commission on the Causes and Prevention of Violence. In R. K. Baker and S. J. Ball (Eds.), *Violence in the Media* (pp. 311–340). Washington, DC: Government Printing Office.

Gesser-Edelsburg, A., Mordini, E., James, J. J., Greco, D., and Green, M. S. (2014a). Risk communication recommendations and implementation during emerging infectious diseases: A case study of the 2009 H1N1 influenza Pandemic . *Disaster Medicine and Public Health Preparedness*, 8(02), 158–169.

Gesser-Edelsburg, A., Shir-Raz, Y., Hayek, S., and Sassoni-Bar Lev, O. (2015). What does the public know about Ebola? The public's risk perceptions regarding the current Ebola outbreak in an as-yet unaffected country. *American Journal of Infection Control*, 43(7), 669–675.

Gesser-Edelsburg, A., Walter, N., and Green, M. S. (2014b). Health care workers – part of the system or part of the public? Ambivalent risk perception in health care workers. *American Journal of Infection Control*, 42(8), 829–833.

Gesser-Edelsburg, A., Walter, N., and Shir-Raz, Y. (2016). The "new public" and the "good ol' press": Evaluating online news sources during the 2013 polio outbreak in Israel. *Health Communication*.

Goldacre, B, (2013). *Bad Pharma: How Drug Companies Mislead Doctors and Harm Patients.* New York: Faber and Faber.

Goldstein, M. A., Goodman, A., del Carmen, M. G., and Wilbur, D. C. (2009). Case 10–2009 – A 23-year-old woman with an abnormal papanicolaou smear. *New England Journal of Medicine*, 360(13), 1337–1344.

Gosden, R., and Beder, S. (2001). Pharmaceutical industry agenda setting in mental health policies. *Ethical Human Sciences and Services*, 3(3), 147–159.

Gunter, B. (2003). *News and the Net.* Mahwah, NJ: Lawrence Erlbaum.

Hachim, M., and Peled-Raz, M. (2007). The vaccine against human papillomavirus (HPV): Should and how can it be integrated into the regular vaccine schedule? *Medicine and Law*, 37, 55–66.

Hagan, S. (2014). Ebola epidemic affects press freedom in West Africa: Report highlights challenge of disseminating accurate, fair information. Vienna: International Press Institute.

Hakim, H., Gaur, A. H., and McCullers, J. A. (2011). Motivating factors for high rates of influenza vaccination among healthcare workers. *Vaccine*, 29(35), 5963–5969.

Hanitzsch, T. (2007). Deconstructing journalism culture: Toward a universal theory. *Communication Theory*, 17(4), 367–385.

Hanitzsch, T. (2011). Populist disseminators, detached watchdogs, critical change agents and opportunist facilitators: Professional milieus, the journalistic field and autonomy in 18 countries. *International Communication Gazette*, 73(6), 477–494.

Hargreaves, I. (2001). Who's misunderstanding whom? The Pantaneto Forum.

Hathaway, J. K. (2012). HPV: diagnosis, prevention, and treatment. *Clinical Obstetrics and Gynecology*, 55(3), 671–680.

Herman, E. S., and Chomsky, N. (1988). *Manufacturing Consent: The Political Economy of the Mass Media*. New York: Pantheon Books.

Hinnant, A., and Len-Ríos, M. E. (2009). Tacit understandings of health literacy: Interview and survey research with health journalists. *Science Communication*, 31(1), 84–115.

Hoffman-Goetz, L., and MacDonald, M. (1999). Cancer coverage in mass-circulating Canadian women's magazines. *Canadian Journal of Public Health*, 90(1), 55–59.

Høye, S., and Hjortdahl, P. (2002). "New wonder pill!"– what do Norwegian newspapers write? *Tidsskrift for den Norske laegeforening: Tidsskrift for Praktisk Medicin, ny Raekke*, 122(17), 1671–1676.

Iaboli, L., Caselli, L., Filice, A., Russi, G., and Belletti, E. (2010). The unbearable lightness of health science reporting: A week examining Italian print media. *PLoS ONE*, 5(3), e9829.

IFJ. (1986). IFJ declaration of principles on the conduct of journalists. Available at: www.ifj.org/about-ifj/ifj-code-of-principles/(accessed May 13, 2016).

Innes, E. (2013). Teacher, 25, died after being diagnosed with cervical cancer just days after attending her first routine smear test . *Daily Mail Online*. June 6,. Available at: www.dailymail.co.uk/health/article-2337033/Teacher-died-cervical-cancer-just-months-routine-smear-test.html#ixzz408lDAaiK

Israel Medical Association Legal Department. (2014). Verdict: Violation of freedom of occupation in front of harm to the public peace. *Harefuah*, January–February, 44–45.

Jackson, S. (2008). Fearing the rise of 'churnalism'. *The Australian*, June 5, p. 33. Available at: www.theaustralian.news.com.au/story/0,,23811929-7582,00.html?from=public_rss

Jemal, A., Center, M. M., DeSantis, C., and Ward, E. M. (2010). Global patterns of cancer incidence and mortality rates and trends. *Cancer Epidemiology, Biomarkers and Prevention*, 19(8), 1893–1907.

Johnson, T. (1998). Medicine and the media. *New England Journal of Medicine*, 339(2), 87–92.

Kenix, L. J. (2013). A converging image? Commercialism and the visual identity of alternative and mainstream news websites. *Journalism Studies*, 14(6), 835–856.

Kirchhoff, S. M. (2009). *The U.S. Newspaper Industry in Transition*. Washington, DC: Congressional Research Service.

Klein, A. (2008). Between myths and science: The AIDS narrative in Israel media 1981–2007 as a case study of cultural constructions of illness. *Media Frames: Israeli Journal of Communication*, 2, 50–85.

Komesaroff, P. A. (2010). Ethical issues associated with gifts provided to physicians by the pharmaceutical industry. *Internal Medicine Journal*, 40(5), 321–322.

Kroll, D. (2014). Dr. Paul Offit: 'journalism jail' for faulty medical reporting. *Forbes*. March 29.

Kua, E., Reder, M., and Grossel, M. J. (2004). Science in the news: A study of reporting genomics. *Public Understanding of Science*, 13(3), 309–322.

Lam, P. P., and McGeer, A. (2011). Communication strategies for the 2009 influenza A (H1N1) pandemic. Available at: http://centreinfection.s3.amazonaws.com/wp/sites/2/2015/04/05205704/H1N1_5_final.pdf (accessed May 14, 2016).

Lariscy, R. W., Avery, E. J., and Sohn, Y. (2010). Health journalists and three levels of public information: Issue and agenda disparities? *Journal of Public Relations Research*, 22(2), 113–135.

Leask, J., Hooker, C., and King, C. (2010). Media coverage of health issues and how to work more effectively with journalists: A qualitative study. *BMC Public Health*, 10, 535.

Len-Ríos, M. E., Hinnant, A., Park, S. A., Cameron, G. T., Frisby, C. M., and Lee, Y. (2009). Health news agenda building: Journalists' perceptions of the role of public relations. *Journalism and Mass Communication Quarterly*, 86(2), 315–331.

Levi, R. (2001). *Medical Journalism: Exposing Fact, Fiction, Fraud*. Ames, IA: Iowa State University Press.

Lewis, J., Williams, A., and Franklin, B. (2008). A compromised fourth estate? *Journalism Studies*, 9(1), 1–20.

Logan, R. A. (1991). Popularization versus secularization: Media coverage of health. In L. Wilkins and P. Patterson (Eds.), *Risky Business: Communicating Issues of Science, Risk, and Public Policy* (pp. 44–59). New York: Greenwood Press.

Lowy, I. (2011). *A Woman's Disease: The History of Cervical Cancer*. Oxford: Oxford University Press.

Mahmud, S. (May 13, 2009). Is the newspaper industry at death's door? Available at: www.mysinchew.com/node/24415?tid=14 (accessed May 13, 2016).

Manovich, L. (2001). *The Language of New Media*. Cambridge, MA: The MIT Press.

McNair, B. (2009). *News and Journalism in the UK* (Fifth edition). London: Routledge.

Media Foundation for West Africa (2014). Special Report on Ebola and free expression in West Africa. Available at: http://mfwa.africafex.org/wp-content/uploads/2015/11/MFWA-Special-Report-on-Ebola-and-Free-Expression-in-West-Africa.pdf

Miranda, G. F., Vercellesi, L., and Bruno, F. (2004). Information sources in biomedical science and medical journalism: Methodological approaches and assessment. *Pharmacological Research*, 50(3), 267–272.

Morgan, M., and Signorielli, N. (1990). Cultivation analysis conceptualization and methodology. In N. Signorielli and M. Morgan (Eds.), *Cultivation Analysis: New Directions in Media Effects Research* (pp. 13–34). Newbury Park, CA: Sage.

Morgan, M. G., Fischhoff, B., Bostrom, A., and Atman, C. J. (2002). *Risk Communication: A Mental Models Approach*. New York:Cambridge University Press.

Morgan, M. G., Fischhoff, B., Bostrom, A., Lave, L., and Atman, C. (1992). ES&T features. Communicating risk to the public. First, learn what people know and believe. *Environmental Science and Technology*, 26(11), 2048–2056.

Moynihan, R., Bero, L., Ross-Degnan, D., *et al.* (2000). Coverage by the news media of the benefits and risks of medications. *New England Journal of Medicine*, 342(22), 1645–1650.

Moynihan, R., Cooke, G. P. E., Doust, J. A., Bero, L., Hill, S., and Glasziou, P. P. (2013). Expanding disease definitions in guidelines and expert panel ties to industry:

A cross-sectional study of common conditions in the United States. *PLoS Medicine*, 10(8), e1001500.

Moynihan, R., and Sweet, M. (2000). Medicine, the media and monetary interests: The need for transparency and professionalism. *The Medical Journal of Australia*, 173(11), 631–634.

National Advisory Committee on Immunization. (2007). Statement on human papillomavirus vaccine. *Canada Communicable Disease Report*, 33(ACS-2).

Nelkin, D. (1995). *Selling Science: How the Press Covers Science and Technology.* New York: W.H. Freeman and Company.

Nelkin, D. (1996). An uneasy relationship: The tensions between medicine and the media. *The Lancet*, 347(9015), 1600–1603.

Norris, P., Herxheimer, A., Lexchin, J., and Mansfield, P. (2004). *Drug Promotion: What We Know, What We Have Yet to Learn-Reviews of Materials in the WHO/ HAI Database on Drug promotion.* EDM research series No. 032. Geneva: World Health Organization and Health Action International.

Obregon, R., and Waisbord, S. (2012). *The Handbook of Global Health Communication.* Malden, MA: Wiley-Blackwell.

*OC Register.* (2011). Corrections for April 18. Available at: www.ocregister.com/arti cles/correction-296910-dated-entitled.html (accessed May 13, 2016).

Oreskes, N., and Conway, E. M. (2011). *Merchants of Doubt: How a Handful of Scientists Obscured the Truth on Issues from Tobacco Smoke to Global Warming.* New York: Bloomsbury Press.

Park, H., and Reber, B. H. (2010). Using public relations to promote health: A framing analysis of public relations strategies among health associations. *Journal of Health Communication*, 15(1), 39–54.

Parkin, D. M. (2006). The global health burden of infection-associated cancers in the year 2002. *International Journal of Cancer*, 118(12), 3030–3044.

Parry, L. (, 2014). Young mother died from cervical cancer after visiting doctors nine times complaining of bloating, tiredness and stomach pain - but was told she was 'too young' to have the disease. *Daily Mail Online*. September 25. Available at: www.dailymail.co.uk/health/article-2767864/My-daughter-died-cervical-cancer-visiting-doctors-NINE-times-Mother-s-campaign-lower-smear-test-age-22-year-old-told-young-screening.html#ixzz42D6RJc77

Pfund, N., and Hofstadter, L. (1981). Biomedical innovation and the press. *Journal of Communication*, 31(2), 138–154.

Piccirillo, B., and Gaeta, T. (2006). Survey on use of and attitudes toward influenza vaccination among emergency department staff in a New York metropolitan hospital. *Infection Control and Hospital Epidemiology*, 27(6), 618–622.

Quandt, T. (2008). (No) news on the world wide web? A comparative content analysis of online news in Europe and the United States. *Journalism Studies*, 9(5), 717–738.

Quinn, S. (2002). *Knowledge Management in the Digital Newsroom.* Oxford: Focal Press.

Rampton, S., and Stauber, J. (2002). *Trust Us We're Experts: How Industry Manipulates Science and Gambles with Your Future.* New York: Jeremy P. Tarcher/ Putnam.

Ransohoff, D. F., and Ransohoff, R. M. (2001). Sensationalism in the media: When scientists and journalists may be complicit collaborators. *Effective Clinical Practice*, 4(4), 185–188.

Rebmann, T., Wright, K. S., Anthony, J., Knaup, R. C., and Peters, E. B. (2012a). Seasonal and H1N1 influenza vaccine compliance and intent to be vaccinated among emergency medical services personnel. *American Journal of Infection Control*, 40(7), 632–636.

Rebmann, T., Wright, K. S., Anthony, J., Knaup, R. C., and Peters, E. B. (2012b). Seasonal influenza vaccine compliance among hospital-based and nonhospital-based healthcare workers. *Infection Control and Hospital Epidemiology*, 33(3), 243–249.

Rorty, R. (1991). *Objectivity, Relativism and Truth: Philosophical Papers*. Cambridge: Cambridge University Press.

Rose, M. (1991). Activism in the 90s: Changing roles for public relations. *Public Relations Quarterly*, 36(3), 28–32.

Rothman, D. J., McDonald, W. J., Berkowitz, C. D., *et al.* (2009). Professional medical associations and their relationships with industry: A proposal for controlling conflict of interest. *JAMA*, 301(13), 1367–1372.

Schiffman, M., and Kjaer, S. K. (2003). Chapter 2: Natural history of anogenital human papillomavirus infection and neoplasia. *Journal of the National Cancer Institute Monographs*, 2003(31), 14–19.

Schwartz, L. M., Woloshin, S., and Moynihan, R. (2008). Who's watching the watchdogs? *BMJ*, 337, a2535.

Schwitzer, G. (1992). The magical medical media tour. *JAMA*, 267(14), 1969–1971.

Schwitzer, G. (2003). How the media left the evidence out in the cold. *BMJ*, 326(7403), 1403–1404.

Schwitzer, G. (2008). How do US journalists cover treatments, tests, products, and procedures? An evaluation of 500 stories. *PLoS Medicine*, 5(5), e95.

Seale, H., Wang, Q., Yang, P., Dwyer, D. E., Wang, X., Zhang, Y., et al. (2010). Influenza vaccination amongst hospital health care workers in Beijing. *Occupational Medicine*, 60(5), 335–339.

Seletzky, M., and Lehman-Wilzig, S. (2010). Factors underlying organizations' successful press release publication in newspapers: Additional PR elements for the evolving "press agentry" and "public information" models. *International Journal of Strategic Communication*, 4(4), 244–266.

Shoemaker, P. J., and Reese, S. D. (1996). *Mediating the Message: Theories of Influences on Mass Media Content* (Vol. 2). White Plains, NY: Longman.

Shuchman, M., and Wilkes, M. S. (1997). Medical scientists and health news reporting: A case of miscommunication. *Annals of Internal Medicine*, 126(12), 976–982.

Singer, J. B. (1997). Still guarding the gate?: The newspaper journalist's role in an on-line world. *Convergence: The International Journal of Research into New Media Technologies*, 3(1), 72–89.

Slovic, P., Finucane, M. L., Peters, E., and MacGregor, D. G. (2004). Risk as analysis and risk as feelings: Some thoughts about affect, reason, risk, and rationality. *Risk Analysis*, 24(2), 311–322.

Smedley, J., Poole, J., Waclawski, E., *et al.* (2007). Influenza immunisation: Attitudes and beliefs of UK healthcare workers. *Occupational and Environmental Medicine*, 64(4), 223–227.

Stocking, S. H., and Holstein, L. W. (1993). Constructing and reconstructing scientific ignorance: Ignorance claims in science and journalism. *Science Communication*, 15(2), 186–210.

Stryker, J., Solky, B. A., and Emmons, K. M. (2005). A content analysis of news coverage of skin cancer prevention and detection, 1979 to 2003. *Archives of Dermatology*, 141(4), 491–496.

Sumner, P., Vivian-Griffiths, S., Boivin, J., *et al.* (2014). The association between exaggeration in health related science news and academic press releases: Retrospective observational study. *BMJ*, 349, g7015.

Takayanagi, I. J., Cardoso, M. R. A., Costa, S. F., Araya, M. E. S., and Machado, C. M. (2007). Attitudes of health care workers to influenza vaccination: Why are they not vaccinated? *American Journal of Infection Control*, 35(1), 56–61.

Thacker, P. D. (, 2015). Where do science journalists draw the line? *Columbia Journalism Review.* November 23. Available at: www.cjr.org/criticism/science_journalism_conflicts_of_interest.php

Tversky, A., and Kahneman, D. (1981). The framing of decisions and the psychology of choice. *Science*, 211(4481), 453–458.

Vasterman, P. L. M., and Ruigrok, N. (2013). Pandemic alarm in the Dutch media: Media coverage of the 2009 influenza A (H1N1) pandemic and the role of the expert sources. *European Journal of Communication*, 28(4), 436–453.

Vírseda, S., Restrepo, M. A., Arranz, E., et al. (2010). Seasonal and pandemic A (H1N1) 2009 influenza vaccination coverage and attitudes among health-care workers in a Spanish university hospital. *Vaccine*, 28(30), 4751–4757.

Vogt, B. (2011). *The Church and New Media: Blogging Converts, Online Activists, and Bishops Who Tweet.* Huntington, IN: Our Sunday Visitor.

Voss, M. (2002). Checking the pulse: Midwestern reporters' opinions on their ability to report health care news. *American Journal of Public Health*, 92(7), 1158–1160.

Weimann, G., and Lev, E. (2006). Mass-mediated medicine. *Israel Medical Association Journal*, 8(11), 757–762.

Weingarten, S., Riedinger, M., Bolton, L. B., Miles, P., and Ault, M. (1989). Barriers to influenza vaccine acceptance A survey of physicians and nurses. *American Journal of Infection Control*, 17(4), 202–207.

Weiss, C. H., and Singer, E. (1988). *Reporting of Social Science in the National Media.* New York: Russell Sage Foundation.

Weitkamp, E. (2014). On the roles of scientists, press officers and journalists. *Journal of Science Communication*, 13(03).

Weitkamp, E., and Eidsvaag, T. (2014). Agenda building in media coverage of food research. *Journalism Practice*, 8(6), 871–886.

WHO. (2009a). Transcript of virtual press conference with Gregory Hartl, WHO Spokesperson for Epidemic and Pandemic Diseases, and Dr Sylvie Briand, Project leader in the Global Influenza Programme, World Health Organization. May 13. Geneva: World Health Organization.

WHO. (2009b). Transcript of virtual press conference with Gregory Hartl, WHO Spokesperson for Epidemic and Pandemic Diseases, and Dr Keiji Fukuda, Assistant Director-General ad Interim for Health Security and Environment. May 26. Geneva: World Health Organization.

WHO. (2009c). Transcript of virtual press conference with Gregory Hartl, WHO Spokesperson for Global Alert and Response and Dr Marie-Paule Kieny, Director of the Initiative for Vaccine Research, World Health Organization. July 13. Geneva: World Health Organization.

WHO. (2009d). Transcript of WHO virtual press conference of 6 August 2009 with Dr Marie-Paule Kieny, Director of the Initiative for Vaccine Research at WHO Headquarters and Gregory Hartl, Spokesperson for H1N1. August 6.Geneva: World Health Organization.

WHO. (2010). Transcript of virtual press conference with Dr Margaret Chan, Director-General, World Health Organization and Dr Keiji Fukuda, Special Adviser to the Director-General on Pandemic Influenza. August 10. Geneva: World Health Organization.

WHO. (2015). Human papillomavirus (HPV) and cervical cancer. Fact sheet N°380. Available at: www.who.int/mediacentre/factsheets/fs380/en/(accessed May 1, 2016).

Wicker, S., Rabenau, H. F., Doerr, H. W., and Allwinn, R. (2009). Influenza vaccination compliance among health care workers in a German university hospital. *Infection*, 37(3), 197–202.

Wicker, S., Rabenau, H. F., Gottschalk, R., Krause, G., and McLennan, S. (2010). Low influenza vaccination rates among healthcare workers. Time to take a different approach. *Bundesgesundheitsblatt Gesundheitsforschung Gesundheitsschutz*, 53(12), 1298–1303.

Wilkins, L. (1987). *Shared Vulnerability: The Media and American Perceptions of the Bhopal Disaster*. New York: Greenwood Press.

Willis, B. C., and Wortley, P. (2007). Nurses' attitudes and beliefs about influenza and the influenza vaccine: A summary of focus groups in Alabama and Michigan. *American Journal of Infection Control*, 35(1), 20–24.

Wilson, P. M., Booth, A. M., Eastwood, A., and Watt, I. S. (2008). Deconstructing media coverage of trastuzumab (Herceptin): An analysis of national newspaper coverage. *Journal of the Royal Society of Medicine*, 101(3), 125–132.

Winsten, J. A. (1985). Science and the media: The boundaries of truth. *Health Affairs*, 4(1), 5–23.

Yap, B. (2009). Time running out for newspapers . *The Malaysian Insider*, June 5. Available at: www.malaysianbar.org.my/general_opinions/comments/time_running_out_for_newspapers.html

Yavchitz, A., Boutron, I., Bafeta, A., Marroun, I., Charles, P., Mantz, J., et al. (2012). Misrepresentation of randomized controlled trials in press releases and news coverage: A cohort study. *PLoS Medicine*, 9(9), e1001308.

Zuckerman, D. (2003). Hype in health reporting: "Checkbook science" buys distortion of medical news. *International Journal of Health Services*, 33(2), 383–389.

# 6 The Public's Understanding and Decision-Making regarding Science and Risk

The term "panic" is rooted in the Greek word *panikon* – "sudden fear." It derives from the name of the Greek god Pan, god of shepherds, flocks, and forests in Greek mythology. According to myth, the feral god (depicted as half-goat, half-man) would often hide in the bushes along a forest trail, and as travelers passed, frighten them by suddenly manifesting himself (Hoffman, 2013). Konstan (2006) explains that irrationality, or the absence of an identifiable cause, is a central characteristic of panic. For example, he cites (Elster, 1999, p. 313), who includes "[p]anics or phobias that lack cognitive support" in a list of "putatively irrational emotions." While today panic is attributed to both groups and individuals, the ancient Greeks understood it as a collective response to a sudden indistinct threat. As Borgeaud (1988, pp. 88–89) concludes:

> Panic is always irrational terror involving noise and confused disturbance that unexpectedly overtakes a military encampment, usually at night. Its suddenness, its immediacy, is stressed ... Furthermore, there is a stress on the lack of any visible cause, a lack that leads to fantasy; the victims of panic are in the grip of imagination, which is to say, of their worst fears. Any noise is immediately taken as the enemy in full attack.

But do panic and irrationality indeed characterize the most widespread public response to disease outbreaks?

## The public's reaction to catastrophes: the panic myth

In February 2016, as the WHO declared that the cluster of Microcephaly and Guillain-Barré syndrome cases reported in Brazil was strongly suspected to be associated with the Zika virus outbreak (WHO, 2016), and predicted that the virus was likely to spread throughout most of the Americas by the end of the year (Miles and Hirschler, 2016), President Obama urged the American public not to panic. "There shouldn't be panic on this. This is not something where people are going to die from it," he said in an interview on *CBS This Morning* (Cohen, 2016). His reassurance came following warnings from the

US Senate Majority Leader Mitch McConnell that the president needed to act quickly, before panic gripped the country as it did when the Ebola virus dominated headlines in 2014. "We need to get out in front of the Zika virus to make sure that we don't end up having the kind of feeling across the country that we're sort of reacting too late, like we did on Ebola," McConnell said (Bolton, 2016).

Indeed, politicians, health officials, experts, and journalists often relate to the public's concerns when facing an emerging disease outbreak, and the desire for more protective policies, in terms of "panic" and "hysteria" (Sandman, 2014). The public's response to the appearance of four Ebola cases in the USA and to the different approaches adopted by various authorities with regard to the precautionary measures that needed to be taken were perceived as a "national panic" (Gonsalves and Staley 2014; Viebeck, 2014). Maryn McKenna (2014) dubbed this response "Ebolanoia." The WHO Pandemic Influenza Risk Management WHO Interim Guidance (WHO, 2013, p. 28) advises governments to "conduct frequent and pre-announced public briefings through popular media outlets such as the web, television, social media and radio *to counter panic and dispel rumors.*" Such advice is based on the assumption that responses such as panic, confusion, and rumors are common in risk situations, and especially when the risks involve uncertainty, such as emerging outbreaks.

Contrary to this widely-accepted view, empiric studies of public response to extreme situations (such as earthquakes, fires, hurricanes) have evinced the opposite findings. As panic expert Lee Clarke notes:

> People rarely panic, at least in the usual sense that word is used. Even when people feel "excessive fear" – a sense of overwhelming doom – they usually avoid "injudicious efforts" and "chaos." In particular, they are unlikely to cause harm to others as they reach for safety and may even put their own lives at risk to help others.
>
> (Clarke, 2002, p. 21)

Clarke argues that in extreme situations the public behaves the same way as it does in everyday life.

> People die the same way they live, with friends, loved ones and colleagues – in communities. When danger arises, the rule – as in normal situations – is for people to help those next to them before they help themselves … Disasters, like other social situations, have rules, and people generally follow them. They are not special rules, even though disasters are special situations. The rules are the same ones at work when the theater is not on fire. Human nature is social, not individually egoistic. People are naturally social, and calamities often strengthen social bonds.
>
> (Clarke, 2002, pp. 24–25)

Norris Johnson, who examined three cases of disasters in which there was a breakdown of social order, examined whether in extreme conditions there is a clash between productive and supportive behavior, on the one hand, and ruthless behavior, on the other. His analysis found no cruel behavior between people occurred because the normative social order still operates under extreme conditions:

> General societal norms continued to constrain individual behavior, and formal roles in groups continued to be performed ... As a result, action was not based on individual concerns alone, but on general civility and a concern for others as well.
>
> (Johnson, 1987, p. 181)

Other studies indicate that in extreme situations people are more likely to react to catastrophes by social cohesion and mutual trust than by demonstrations of panic (Erikson, 1994).

## Using panic as an excuse for lack of transparency

As several scholars have pointed out, the "panic assumption" often leads organizations and governments to refrain from communicating risks (Maxim et al., 2013; Sandman, 2006; Sjöberg, 1998). Furthermore, even when the risk is exposed, often through the social media, and its communication becomes unavoidable, experts and organizations are often afraid to reveal all of the available information and prefer to provide a straightforward and unambiguous explanation.

Policy makers use panic as an excuse to hide, avoid sharing, and even deny information, arguing that the public will not be able to handle it (Clarke, 2002).

Sometimes leaders, claiming to pre-empt public panic, overpromise safety (Clarke, 1999). Likewise, people sometimes worry and express anxiety not because of their natural inclination to panic but as a result of the authorities' helplessness and failure to create a sense of trust, especially caused by misrepresentation.

The lack of responsible and effective management by the authorities has constituted a problem throughout the course of human history. In his book *Cultures of Plague: Medical Thinking at the End of the Renaissance*, Cohn Jr. (2010) describes how during the 1575–1578 plague outbreak in Italy, descriptions of mass fear and panic became increasingly widespread. Physicians from that period who attempted to understand why the poor were more likely to contract the disease than wealthier classes and why it spread mostly in poor neighborhoods, pointed out that the lower classes invested great efforts in concealing the disease, for fear of being refused treatment by doctors and of being abandoned by relatives, and that the little property they owned would be burnt. Additional reasons that accounted for the spread of the disease were the inadequate provisioning of necessary needs, doctors' lack of experience, and the failure of governors to clean the streets and remove filth, and to supply medications and medical treatment, especially to the poor. Thus, the fear that took hold was far from irrational or unfounded, and was in fact mainly a response to flawed health policies and the incompetence of governments.

The interesting paradox that this issue raises is that when it comes to motivating the public to comply with policies, the organizations do not hesitate to instigate worry and anxiety among the public, and even see this practice as vital, as Glen Nowak, the former CDC media relations director, stated in his 2004 presentation (Nowak, 2004). "And can leave you searching for the 'Holy Grail' of Health Communication," Nowak added, ridiculing Lanard and Sandman's article from that same year (March 25; Lanard and Sandman, 2004), which urged organizations not to over-diagnose or over-plan for panic in crisis situations, and not to over-reassure the public. "The belief that you can inform and warn people, and get them to take appropriate actions or precautions with respect to a health threat or risk without actually making them anxious or concerned ... This is not possible." Nowak rejected Lanard and Sandman's recommendations. "Rather ... This is like breaking up with your boyfriend without hurting his feelings. It can't be done."

The authorities' dual tendency to cite panic as a reason for not providing straightforward and full information, on one hand, and on the other hand, to deliberately engender that panic leads, as we have shown (in Chapter 4), to the increasing and sometimes unfounded strategy of intimidation. Is there a basis for the belief that in order to motivate people to action you cannot transmit information without making them anxious or creating panic?

## How do people make decisions during a crisis? And what do people want from the authorities?

Slovic et al. (2004) have explored the association between the analytical and emotional aspects of risk perception, specifically the association between analytical risk analysis and experience-based risk perception. They describe the "analytical system" as a person's ability to analyze rules and norms and calculate risks and opportunities, whereas the "experiential system" is intuitive, quick, automatic and partially subconscious. Studies assessing the public's risk perceptions deal alternately with the analytical and experiential aspects.

Decision-making in risk situations is the result of a combination of experience, knowledge, and affect. Affect is very significant in the decision-making process. Alhakami and Slovic (1994) found that the inverse relationship between perceived risk and perceived benefit of an activity is linked to the strength of positive or negative affect associated with that activity. This result implies that people's judgments are based not only on what they think about something, but also on how they feel about it. The process of the "affect heuristic" suggests that if a general affective view guides perceptions of risk and benefit, then perception regarding risk can be changed (affected) by receiving information about benefit – and vice versa.

The question is how the authorities deal with the emotional component. How do they build a relationship with the public that will elicit positive affect? Some decision-makers tend to ignore the affective dimension or use it as a threat.

As in any human relationship, trust is built on what a person thinks about the risk communicator and what the communicator feels towards them. In studies that tested the effectiveness of risk communication in the doctor–patient relationship, it was found that the emotional component played a key role.

Slovic, Peters, Finucane, and Macgregor (2005) opined that patients and doctors must often make decisions in environments with high levels of affect (at least for the patient) and vulnerability. Therefore, the doctor–patient dialog and its consequences are also informed by affect (Gregory et al., 2011).

If we apply the analogy of the doctor–patient relationship to the relationship between the health officials and the general public, it is important for the relationship to be based on empathy and a positive emotional relationship in order for there to be trust when an epidemic crisis occurs.

Furthermore, the authorities' tendency to cultivate the public's fears and concerns, without empowering their self-efficacy, contradicts the theory of the Extended Parallel Process Model (EPPM) (Witte, 1994), which attempts to predict how individuals react when confronted with fear-inducing stimuli. In order for fear-based policies to be effective, they must induce a moderate level of fear and a higher level of self-efficacy and response efficacy. When the public feels that there is a higher level of fear than efficacy, the message is ineffective.

In general, studies indicate that the public wants full transparency of information. When people become aware of a risk, if they feel they do not have sufficient information about it, this can increase their sense of uncertainty and negative feelings (Gesser-Edelsburg, Shir-Raz and Green, 2016; Griffin et al., 1999; Huurne and Gutteling, 2008; Kahlor, 2010). This is especially true in situations where the risk is perceived as severe and uncontrollable (Witte, 1992). Communicating risks and giving sufficient information do not produce negative reactions among the public in terms of behavior. On the contrary, it can help mitigate negative feelings (De Vocht et al., 2016; Lofstedt, 2006; Palenchar and Heath, 2002; Slovic, 1991).

Health authorities often argue that even though the public demands full and complete information, lay people are really unable to understand complex health information, and would actually prefer for the authorities to instruct them on how and when to act.

## The public's attitude towards science in the decision-making process

For years, it was believed that there was a gap between experts and the public in the way they understand and want information and in the way they think about science.

The mental models approach (Morgan et al., 2002) indicates a distinction between experts and the public, concluding that it is necessary to understand how the public thinks in order to shape risk communication messages and in order to address gaps or inconsistencies in the public's knowledge.

We believe that the assumption that professionals have greater expertise than the public needs to be reconsidered. What is implied by the term "experts"? Aside from professionals who specialize in the scientific issue at hand, does this category also include public officials? We would like to suggest that there is a difference between experts (who specialize in a particular subject for their entire professional life) and public health professionals, who are often considered experts by the authorities, themselves and even the public. Studies have found that despite their public image as experts, healthcare professionals are no different from the average citizen in terms of their anxieties and also in terms of their knowledge. For instance, studies that examined public health workers' vaccination compliance found that many barriers influence their lack of compliance with vaccination even though they are a "professional" public (Heimberger et al., 1995; Marshall, 2013). Studies of healthcare workers have found that their hesitations regarding vaccinations are similar to those of the rest of the public, which is concerned about side effects, the novelty of the vaccination, and lack of faith in its efficacy and the severity of the disease (Smedley et al., 2007).

One such study that we noted earlier in the chapter on health workers was a comparative examination of public health workers and the general public regarding their risk perception in light of the emerging Avian Influenza A (H7N9) in China in 2013. This study, conducted by Gesser-Edelsburg, Walter, and Green (2014), found that public health professionals' risk analysis was the same as the general public's. When risk perception is relatively low, healthcare professionals tended to base their attitudes toward vaccines on analytical knowledge, whereas in situations with high risk perception, the results did not indicate any significant difference between Israeli health professionals and the Israeli general public. Both groups based their attitudes more on emotions and personal experience than on analytical knowledge.

Another erroneous perception regarding authorities is the perception that the public does not have the capability to understand scientific uncertainty and therefore needs to be given clear instructions and simple messages. We believe that this perception also stems from the gap between the experts and the public. This perception is expressed by the Information Deficit Model (Dickson, 2005), which distinguishes between experts who have the information and non-experts who lack information and understanding, and are in some way ignorant of the scientific knowledge about risk and probability.

Research has shown that every subpopulation has a different level of health literacy and therefore needs to have information tailored to their conceptual and cultural level. Tailoring information does not entail giving partial or selective information – instead, it refers to how full information should be conveyed in a thoughtful way. However, this has been used as a basis for the erroneous perception that segments of the public cannot comprehend any level of scientific complexity and must therefore be given partial or simplified information.

Irwin's concept of Citizen Science (Irwin, 1995) undermined the claim that the public needs simplistic and clear explanations, by showing that the dualistic paradigm of an ignorant public versus knowledgeable experts is no longer relevant or has been updated. In the technological climate of the 21st century, there are diverse voices and perspectives on knowledge, rather than one monolithic knowledge. The public understands science differently in diverse contexts and in different social groups.

Studies we conducted over the last few years on a range of subjects have tended to support Irwin's argument. We conducted a case study during the Ebola epidemic on the topic of Hickox, the nurse who was quarantined in October 2014 at a New Jersey hospital upon her return to the USA after treating Ebola patients in Sierra Leone. Our study of the Hickox quarantine incident found that both supporters and objectors of the quarantining policy resorted to scientific arguments (Gesser-Edelsburg and Shir-Raz, 2015). This shows that each side understands scientific evidence differently. This refutes the framing by the mainstream U.S. media that those who supported quarantine were "irrational" and fear-driven, whereas those who opposed quarantine and supported Hickox's position were science-based. Moreover, those who opposed quarantine cannot be represented as scientifically-based as opposed to purportedly "irrational" quarantine supporters. Significantly, both sides employed scientific evidence and analyzed the situation according to risk perceptions based on knowledge and common sense.

Another study that we conducted on the Israeli public's reaction to the polio crisis in Israel examined why a population that usually vaccinates its children decided not to vaccinate their children in this crisis. The study revealed that this noncompliance stemmed pre-emininently from the Health Ministry's nonscientific communication (Gesser-Edelsburg, Shir-Raz and Green, 2016).

The Health Ministry's campaign had assumed that in order to motivate parents to get their children vaccinated, they needed to claim almost zero risk.

> The findings indicate that claiming there is no risk whatsoever was inter-preted as neither respecting the public nor credible, and as such, it raised the resistance of those who were deliberating and caused a boomerang effect (Hovland, Janis, and Kelley, 1953).
>
> (Gesser-Edelsburg, Shir-Raz and Green, 2016, p. 421)

In another case study we conducted on the 2013 polio crisis, we examined the sources of information used in new media platforms to determine whether the new media changed the ways we communicate about health issues (Gesser-Edelsburg, Walter and Shir-Raz, 2016). Beyond the differences between various platforms, we found that online information platforms where many laypeople write and express themselves rely not only on popular or pseudoscientific sour-ces, but also on high-quality information. In fact, the analysis indicated that news websites, forums, blogs and Facebook posts offer a unique blend of information, from sources including scientific literature, medical professionals, government representatives, along with pseudoscientific research.

These findings indicate the changing role of citizen journalism. The public's role in the public sphere has transformed from consumer to become more of a partner. The general public now shares the domain that previously belonged to professional journalists. The virtual realm has become more pluralistic and diverse, creating a space for diverse voices from many segments of the population. Participatory or citizen journalism is a grassroots phenomenon, allowing diverse voices and perspectives to be heard.

Numerous online projects have been created to promote so-called public science, based on the understanding that the public can gather information, read about science and make decisions. Many centers of participatory research have been established, such as the Public Science Project (http://publicsciencep roject.org/) and the Society for Participation, Engagement, Action and Knowledge (www.speaksoc.org/). These have become platforms for the general public that has increasingly chosen – as a collective unit – to gather and manage the information it needs, rather than relying only on the authorities.

Critics have argued that the Internet revolution has given rise to shallowness and unprofessionalism. They also claim that citizens will always be outsiders to the system and will never actively participate in decision-making (*The Digital Journalist*, 2009). Contrary to these arguments, those who support citizen journalism maintain that the professionals are misreading the new media and criticizing it from the perspective of the old and conservative media. As Shirky (2002) has argued, "Media people often criticize the content on the internet for being unedited, because everywhere one looks, there is low quality – bad writing, ugly images, poor design." Yet, he claims, they fail to understand that the internet is indeed edited, but in a different way from what they are used to. "Google edits web pages by aggregating user judgment about them, Slashdot edits posts by letting readers rate them, and of course users edit all the time, by choosing what (and who) to read" (Shirky, 2002).

At any rate, research on the quality of citizen journalism's sources and its impact is still in its infancy. Judging it will be possible only when additional empirical studies and comprehensive analyses become available. But we can already claim that the technological revolution has changed the boundaries of the discourse and has led to greater public involvement and activism both before and during epidemic crises.

## References

Alhakami, A. S., and Slovic, P. (1994). A psychological study of the inverse relationship between perceived risk and perceived benefit. *Risk Analysis*, 14(6), 1085–1096.

Bolton, A. (February 2, 2016). McConnell presses Obama to fight Zika virus . *The Hill*. Available at :http://thehill.com/policy/healthcare/267919-mcconnell-presses-obama-to-fight-zika-virus

Borgeaud, P. (1988). *The Cult of Pan in Ancient Greece* (trans. K. Atlass and J. Redfield). Chicago: The University of Chicago Press.

Clarke, L. (1999). *Mission Improbable: Using Fantasy Documents to Tame Disaster.* Chicago: University of Chicago Press.

Clarke, L. (2002). Panic: Myth or reality? *Contexts,* 1(3), 21–26.

Cohen, K. (2016). Obama: Don't 'panic' over the Zika virus . *Washington Examiner,* February 8. Available at: www.washingtonexaminer.com/obama-dont-panic-over-the-zika-virus/article/2582713

Cohn Jr, S. K. (2010). *Cultures of Plague: Medical Thinking at the End of the Renaissance.* Oxford: Oxford University Press.

De Vocht, M., Claeys, A. S., Cauberghe, V., Uyttendaele, M., and Sas, B. (2016). Won't we scare them? The impact of communicating uncontrollable risks on the public's perception. *Journal of Risk Research,* 19(3), 316–330.

Dickson, D. (2005). The case for a 'deficit model' of science communication. *SciDevNet,* June 27.

Elster, J. (1999). *Alchemies of the Mind: Rationality and the Emotions.* Cambridge: Cambridge University Press.

Erikson, K. (1994). *New Species of Trouble: Explorations in Disaster, Trauma, and Community.* New York: W.W. Norton and Co.

Gesser-Edelsburg, A., and Shir-Raz, Y. (2015). Science vs. fear: The Ebola quarantine debate as a case study that reveals how the public perceives risk. *Journal of Risk Research,* Ahead of Print, 1–23.

Gesser-Edelsburg, A., Shir-Raz, Y., and Green, M. S. (2016). Why do parents who usually vaccinate their children hesitate or refuse? General good vs. individual risk. *Journal of Risk Research,* 19(4), 405–424.

Gesser-Edelsburg, A., Walter, N., and Green, M. S. (2014). Health care workers – part of the system or part of the public? Ambivalent risk perception in health care workers. *American Journal of Infection Control,* 42(8), 829–833.

Gesser-Edelsburg, A., Walter, N., and Shir-Raz, Y. (2016). The "new public" and the "good ol' press": Evaluating online news sources during the 2013 polio outbreak in Israel. *Health Communication.*

Gonsalves , G., and Staley , P. (2014). Panic, paranoia, and public health – The AIDS epidemic's lessons for Ebola. *New England Journal of Medicine,* 371(25), 2348–2349.

Gregory, R., Peters, E., and Slovic, P. (2011). Making decisions about prescription drugs: A study of doctor–patient communication. *Health, Risk and Society,* 13(4), 347–371.

Griffin, R. J., Dunwoody, S., and Neuwirth, K. (1999). Proposed model of the relationship of risk information seeking and processing to the development of preventive behaviors. *Environmental Research,* 80(2), S230–S245.

Heimberger, T., Chang, H. G., Shaikh, M., Crotty, L., Morse, D., and Birkhead, G. (1995). Knowledge and attitudes of healthcare workers about influenza: Why are they not getting vaccinated? *Infection Control and Hospital Epidemiology,* 16(7), 412–415.

Hoffman, R. (October 4, 2013). The origin of "panic." Available at: http://drhoffman.com/article/the-origin-of-panic-3/ (accessed May 14, 2016).

Hovland, C. I., Janis, I. L., and Kelley, H. H. (1953). *Communication and Persuasion: Psychological Studies of Opinion Change.* New Haven, CT: Yale University Press.

Huurne, E. T., and Gutteling, J. (2008). Information needs and risk perception as predictors of risk information seeking. *Journal of Risk Research*, 11(7), 847–862.

Irwin, A. (1995). *Citizen Science: A Study of People, Expertise and Sustainable Development*. London: Routledge.

Johnson, N. R. (1987). Panic and the breakdown of social order: Popular myth, social theory, empirical evidence. *Sociological Focus*, 20(3), 171–183.

Kahlor, L. (2010). PRISM: A planned risk information seeking model. *Health Communication*, 25(4), 345–356.

Konstan, D. (2006). *The Emotions of the Ancient Greeks: Studies in Aristotle and Classical Literature*. Toronto: University of Toronto Press.

Lanard, J., and Sandman, P. M. (2004). Four kinds of risk communication in community outreach. Paper presented at the Environmental Public Health Tracking Conference, Philadelphia, PA, March 25.

Lofstedt, R. E. (2006). How can we make food risk communication better?: Where are we and where are we going? *Journal of Risk Research*, 9(8), 869–890.

Marshall, R. J. (2013). Influenza vaccine use among health care workers: Social marketing, policy, and ethics. *Social Marketing Quarterly*, 19(4), 222–229.

Maxim, L., Mansier, P., and Grabar, N. (2013). Public reception of scientific uncertainty in the endocrine disrupter controversy: The case of male fertility. *Journal of Risk Research*, 16(6), 677–695.

McKenna, M. (2014). Ebolanoia: The only thing we have to fear is Ebola itself. *Wired*, October 22.

Miles, T., and Hirschler, B. (2016). Zika virus set to spread across Americas, spurring vaccine hunt. *Reuters*, January 25. Available at: www.reuters.com/article/us-health-zika-idUSKCN0V30U6

Morgan, M. G., Fischhoff, B., Bostrom, A., and Atman, C. J. (2002). *Risk Communication: A Mental Models Approach*. New York: Cambridge University Press.

Nowak, G. (2004). Planning for the 2004–2005 influenza vaccination season: A communication situation analysis. Available at: www.fisique.ca/documents/CDC_2004_flu_nowak.pdf (accessed May 1, 2016).

Palenchar, M. J., and Heath, R. L. (2002). Another part of the risk communication model: Analysis of communication processes and message content. *Journal of Public Relations Research*, 14(2), 127–158.

Sandman, P. M. (2006). Crisis communication best practices: Some quibbles and additions. *Journal of Applied Communication Research*, 34(3), 257–262.

Sandman, P. M. (2014). Ebola in the U.S. (so far): The public health establishment and the quarantine debate, November 15. Available at: www.psandman.com/col/Ebola-4.htm (accessed May 14, 2016).

Shirky, C. (2002). Broadcast institutions, community values. September 9. Available at: www.shirky.com

Sjöberg, L. (1998). Worry and risk perception. *Risk Analysis*, 18(1), 85–93.

Slovic, P. (1991). Beyond numbers: A broader perspective on risk perception and risk communication. In D. G. Mayo and R. D. Hollander (Eds.), *Acceptable Evidence: Science and Values in Risk Management* (pp. 48–65). New York: Oxford University Press.

Slovic, P., Finucane, M. L., Peters, E., and MacGregor, D. G. (2004). Risk as analysis and risk as feelings: Some thoughts about affect, reason, risk, and rationality. *Risk Analysis*, 24(2), 311–322.

Slovic, P., Peters, E., Finucane, M. L., and MacGregor, D. G. (2005). Affect, risk, and decision making. *Health Psychology*, 24(4 Suppl), S35–40.

Smedley, J., Poole, J., Waclawski, E., Stevens, A., Harrison, J., Watson, J., et al. (2007). Influenza immunisation: Attitudes and beliefs of UK healthcare workers. *Occupational and Environmental Medicine*, 64(4), 223–227.

The *Digital Journalist* (2009). Editorial. Let's abolish the term 'citizen journalists'. *The Digital Journalist*, December. Available at: http://digitaljournalist.org/issue0912/lets-abolish-citizen-journalists.html

Viebeck, E. (2014). Health officials struggle to control the media narrative about Ebola. *The Hill*. October 12. Available at: http://thehill.com/policy/healthcare/220458-feds-struggle-to-control-the-media-narrative-about-ebola

WHO. (2013). *Pandemic Influenza Risk Management: WHO Interim Guidance (No. WHO/HSE/HEA/HSP/2013.3)*. Geneva: World Health Organization.

WHO. (2016). WHO Director-General summarizes the outcome of the Emergency Committee regarding clusters of microcephaly and Guillain-Barré syndrome. Available at: www.who.int/mediacentre/news/statements/2016/emergency-committee-zika-microcephaly/en/ (accessed May 14, 2016).

Witte, K. (1992). Putting the fear back into fear appeals: The extended parallel process model. *Communication Monographs*, 59(4), 329–349.

Witte, K. (1994). Fear control and danger control: A test of the extended parallel process model (EPPM). *Communication Monographs*, 61(2), 113–134.

# 7  Observations and Lessons

## Managing health risks in the age of digital media

There is a close interaction between the concepts of power, knowledge and discourse in human society. The philosophers Nietzsche, Derrida, Bourdieu, and Foucault discussed, each in their own way, the materialization of power in discourse. They argued that discourse is based on a logocentric hierarchy that has a center and margins, and that this logocentricity is closely associated with the construction of all of the concepts of absolute truth known to us. According to Foucault (1981), scientific discourse is no different from other forms of discourse, and is context-, time-, and place-dependent. States of illness and health have biological reality, but are measured by their social and cultural contexts. Nonetheless, human societies believe that the knowledge they have is reality itself. This misconception leads people, including experts, to think about the world and identify processes in certain terms, but at the same time it prevents them from noticing details or scientific theories that are inconsistent with the prevailing concepts. Foucault discusses the scientific theory of Gregor Mendel (1822–1884), known as the father of genetics, but who was rejected by the scientists of his time. What Mendel asserted was correct, but his scientific discovery did not fit "within the truth of the biological discourse" of his time (Foucault, 1981, p. 61). Therefore, Foucault distinguishes between "the physical world," and its representation in the scientific theories that translate knowledge into concepts, which become accepted by the public. The acceptance of a theory normalizes the knowledge and makes it "natural." Governmental institutions rule through the normalization of knowledge for the public. According to Foucault, the most effective power ever exercised in modern Western history to date was expressed precisely in the Western capitalist era, in the sense that power became more elusive and obscure than in totalitarian or communist regimes. The middle class gave rise to productive people who, unbeknownst to them, are actually the establishment's agents of persuasion (Mills, 2003). In fact, the politicization of science has been immanent throughout the history of science. Barak Obama, speaking in his first term as President of the USA at the National Academy of Sciences, expressed the way governments use science to realize their interests. "We have watched as scientific integrity has been undermined and scientific research politicized in an effort to advance predetermined ideological agendas" (The White House, 2009).

However, along with the forces trying to use science in the service of economic and political interests, many other forces are trying to free science of those interests. These forces have even succeeded in establishing a wide scientific consensus on various issues, relying on cumulative studies conducted purely for the public's benefit and health (Oreskes and Conway, 2011). In the technological Internet sphere, there have been many changes in the field of knowledge. Two essential changes are the death of exclusivity and the advent of social networks. The death of exclusivity means that knowledge ceased to be the exclusive property of the scientific and industrial communities alone. Many other players have entered the arena, including various subpopulations, who have turned into communities of knowledge in various ways, as discussed in other chapters of this book. The social networks that gave rise to numerous conversations between individuals and groups have created a decentralization and distribution of knowledge in the public sphere between health organizations and the public.

Chapter 1 of this book, which discussed the public sphere and health communication in the context of emergent infectious diseases, presented a framework (see Figure 1.1 in Chapter 1) of a new bifurcated social sphere. The framework emphasized that different elements overlap because communication does not have clear-cut limits: formal stakeholders are not at the center of this model, but rather encompass (and constitute part of) the public. Figure 1.1 illustrates the transformation of the public from recipient to equal partner. For health organizations to deal effectively with Internet decentralization and bifurcation before and after epidemics, they need to metaphorically embrace the public sphere and its collective memory without attempting to dictate to the public unilaterally.

In order to turn that metaphoric embrace into practical directives for health organizations in the virtual age, this chapter underlines the challenges in scientific discourse and possible solutions. Our rationale is that the virtual sphere cannot be approached before we discuss the way the organizations manage scientific discourse. The second part of this chapter presents the challenges of scientific discourse in the technological sphere and suggests possible directions.

## Challenges in the scientific discourse

In his book, *The Wisdom of Crowds: Why the Many Are Smarter Than the Few*, James Surowiecki advocates for the scientific ethos (Surowiecki, 2005). He argues that cooperation and competition can thrive only thanks to the scientific ethos that demands open access to information. Scientists strive to share their knowledge with colleagues, so that it is no longer private property. This turns the public into a partner in the pursuit of knowledge and discovery.

Surowiecki further argues that science depends not only on an ever-growing pool of joint knowledge, but also on trust in the collective ability of the scientific community to distinguish between credible hypotheses and those that lack credibility.

We suggest that in order to create a credible scientific discourse, certain patterns that are still ingrained in the health organizations must be overcome: (1) homogeneous executive committees; (2) public health experts versus "people with agendas"; (3) from certainty to uncertainty; (4) the preference for consensus; (5) conflicts of interest; (6) facts/rationality v. emotions/myths; and (7) the medicalization of public health.

## Homogeneous executive committees

In health ministries throughout the world and their advisory boards there is often a hierarchical structure, where a group of selected experts decides on most of the policy. The same experts often resurface on different advisory boards. What such boards have in common is often the preference for experts from a certain field, without space for ideological or professional diversity. *The Wisdom of Crowds: Why the Many Are Smarter Than the Few* convincingly argues that such wisdom cannot exist in a small group without a diversity of opinions (Surowiecki, 2005). Karen Jehn and her colleagues at the Wharton School (Jehn, 1995), who conducted studies on diversity, conflict and group performance, note that when there is a problem and the solution involves a high level of creativity, then controversy and even conflict in the group lead to better results. Diverse and rich information become decisive factors.

Many studies have shown that in small groups there is usually a tendency to delegitimize or downplay contradictory or new information. New messages are either interpreted as consistent with the old messages, are not fully understood, or are rejected. This is problematic mainly in light of the fact that sometimes information that appears to be marginal or unfounded can turn out to most important. Furthermore, in small groups, there tends to be a structural hierarchy, wherein members accommodate themselves to the chairperson or opinion leader, and those whose views differ avoid voicing their opinions altogether. The absence of intellectual diversity sometimes leads to erroneous conclusions that can have a serious impact on public health.

Jehn finds that if group members try to use force and aspire to reach agreement and consensus, they will "squelch the creativity needed to complete non-routine tasks effectively, because members will focus on building consensus rather than entertaining innovative ideas" (Jehn, 1995, p. 260). Furthermore, studies show that difficulties arise in groups when minority opinion is not voiced because members of the minority group choose to remain silent and avoid conflict (Loury, 1994). They refrain from sharing information with the whole group for various reasons, whether because of conformism or personal conflicts or disputes over the process (Jehn et al., 1999). This can result in "hidden profiles" – important information that is not shared within the group

(Baron and Kerr, 2003). As a result, group members often have information but do not share it, and this can lead to problematic decisions.

Surowiecki discusses this argument in *The Wisdom of Crowds: Why the Many Are Smarter Than the Few*, devoting an entire chapter to an analysis of the Space Shuttle Columbia disaster. In his fascinating analysis he indicates that despite the complex and ramified structure of NASA, which is based on subcommittees, NASA still managed the project hierarchically. The NASA management team ignored the evidence brought to it that could have significantly improved the chances for the Columbia crew to survive. Linda Ham, who headed the operation, and her colleagues on the executive committee, acted like a small group, where the group members assented with their colleagues, and when new and conflicting information arrived at different stages, they treated it as unimportant.

### Public health experts versus "people with agendas"

One of the tobacco industry's most effective strategies was personal attacks on scientists and experts who presented findings that undermined the industry. Such scientists or experts were described as eccentric, marginal, or as "people with agendas." This strategy of personal attack has been used in other industries, and is sometimes also adopted by public health professionals or policy-makers, who attack those who criticize them, and describe them as "people with agendas" or ideologues with research biases. It is misleading to frame opponents as ideologues who stand out from members of the establishment and the scientists who serve it. As the constructivist approach has shown, all scientists without exception have particular values, and the question is whether they are self-reflective and allow their research findings to lead them on a course of exploration and discovery. Furthermore, as Oreskes and Conway (2011) argued in their book, in the context of climate change, the physicists who represented the industry's interests and accused their opponents of having agendas and ideologies turned out to themselves harbor anti-Communist values and openly opposed any government intervention and regulation in the USA:

> Seitz, Jastrow, Nierenberg and Singer had access to power – all the way to the White House – by virtue of their positions as physicists who had won the Cold War. They used their power to support their political agenda, even though it meant attacking science and their fellow scientists, evidently believing that their larger end justified their means.
>
> (Oreskes and Conway, 2011, pp. 213–214)

### From certainty to uncertainty

Although we cannot achieve scientific certainty regarding epidemics, health organizations still tend to frame issues under dispute as certainties. For instance, in the dispute over the modes of transmission of the Ebola virus, most of the experts claimed it was transferred through body fluids, but there were some who claimed it was transferred by air. There is also uncertainty regarding the transmission channel of the Zika virus. The desire for broad scientific consensus is understandable, because it is needed to design policy and promote behavior change. But we believe that a problem arises when scientific disputes are silenced or dismissed in the decision-making process. This occurred, for example, in the case of the HPV vaccine, which has become a routine vaccine in Israel despite the dispute it fomented. The illusion held by the public and some of the experts that there is certainty in science leads to the assumption that if there is uncertainty, it is a sign that the research is incomplete, biased, or problematic. The aspiration of the positivists for "perfection" is not realistic and can create the illusion that if a causal relationship has not been proven beyond the shadow of a doubt, the policy cannot be pursued.

### Preference for consensus

It has been assumed that scientific consensus is the only way to establish science. A common argument is that an idea becomes scientific truth only when the absolute majority of scientists accept it. This argument is frequently made by science historians. One of the reasons for striving to reach scientific consensus is the desire to block doubters with economic and political interests, who try to sow confusion and fears in the minds of the public. We suggest that striving towards consensus can lead to overlooking a minority opinion or a groundbreaking "marginal study." After all, the most significant breakthroughs in science were advanced by rebellious scientists who paved a new way. Furthermore, sometimes the atmosphere within the policy-maker committees is one of silencing opposition under the guise of scientific consensus, with the majority silencing minority opinions that contradict their positions. Moreover, in their media campaigns, health organizations do not mention minority opinions, on the grounds that this would confuse the public. The denial, disregard, or dismissal of minority opinions can elicit public mistrust, since the public wants to be fully informed of all available information.

### Conflicts of interest

The relation between scientists, healthcare professionals, regulators, and industry has been discussed in this book. We noted that conflicts of interest arose during crises or epidemics when officials from health organizations promoted a policy out of economic or political considerations. Conflicts of interest among experts have been widely discussed in academic forums, in the U.S. Congress and in the press. But exposing conflicts of interest is still a prolonged process or a prolonged struggle. Commercial and economic considerations often outweigh scientific considerations under the guise of "science." Many regulators serve the interests of the corporations they over-see. Furthermore, in order to lay the groundwork, doctors and experts present themselves to the public as independent or as the representatives of indepen-dent organizations or websites, while they are actually "astroturfing" – a strategy of hiding the sponsors who stand behind them (Lyon and Maxwell, 2004). Governments themselves often use this strategy, which comes from industry. For example, an ECDC document on how to engage the public by creating a Facebook page, said that the health organization was not officially identified with the site, which was managed by a behind-the-scenes manager. This undermines transparency (ECDC, 2012).

### Facts/rationality vs. emotions/myths

Health organizations often portray opinions or questions that arise from the public as "irrational" or "emotional," which oppose the correct positions, which are the "facts." This dichotomous division contradicts studies (i.e. Kahneman, Slovic, Fischhof, and others) we have cited throughout this book regarding the decision-making process of the public and of experts. This attitude creates a false reality in which the public's questions, worries, concerns or criticism are not given any scientific clout. The problem with such thinking is that it not only deepens the gap between the public and the decision-makers, but it also turns the dialog with health organizations, despite their good intentions, into a dichotomous dispute (true vs. false), rather than allowing an open scientific exchange.

### The medicalization of public health

Vaccines have revolutionized the realm of epidemics. Their contribution to public health is crucial and tangible. But alongside this scientific contribution, organizations have neglected to educate the public in hygiene and scientific literacy. Health organizations seldom initiate discussions of questions and dilemmas about viruses and their significance. Risk communication campaigns turn into vaccine encouragement campaigns, to the point that it is almost impossible to distinguish between government and industry campaigns.

## Suggestions for change

To address these problems and challenges, we suggest the following changes in the organizations' scientific discourse.

### Professionally and intellectually diverse boards

Advisory and executive boards should include professionals from diverse dis-ciplines who maintain different and preferably conflicting positions, in order to conduct meaningful discussions. Diverse, non-hierarchical groups composed of people who do not know each other well are most likely to yield the best results for the organization. Likewise, decision-makers should also consult professionals who are not on the standard advisory boards but outside of the institutional circle, in order to receive diverse input.

Consulting external committees and including experts from diverse disciplines with different ways of thinking should not only be pursued at times of crisis but should be integrated into the routine daily management of health systems' decisions about vaccines and infectious diseases.

### Presenting the consensus alongside minority positions

The establishment's tendency to dismiss dissenting or unpopular opinions and to frame those who express them as eccentric or having "agendas" is problematic not only on the ethical and public levels, but also on the scientific level. In addition to presenting the consensus, health organizations should also present scientific disputes but it is based on credible research that is not driven by conflicts of interest. An integrated presentation of all of the existing knowledge by health organizations can provide the public with a well-rounded picture of the issue, and at the same time give the organizations intellectual flexibility when they seek to discuss complex issues. In Cass Sunstein's book, *Why Societies Need Dissent* (2003), he emphasizes the importance of dispute for maintaining democratic values. Conformism might lead to cognitive and behavioral errors, whereas pluralism allows free thought, tolerance, and the promotion of civil values in a modern country. He claims there is a paradox in which conformism is viewed as protecting societal values, while "dissidents tend to be seen as selfish individualists, embarking on projects of their own. But in an important sense, the opposite is closer to the truth" (Sunstein, 2003, p. 6). Sunstein indicates the importance of cognitive variance and controversy in all areas of life, from sports to decision-making by the White House and the Supreme Court. It is important for people to be exposed to different and varied opinions when making a decision. Most people come to discussions with predispositions, and must be exposed to controversial opinions.

If we apply Sunstein's theory to the health context, dispute can challenge policy makers' decisions especially during epidemic crises, and raise questions and dilemmas that are significant for creating guidelines both for the various systems and for different parts of the public. The tendency to conformism on the part of decision-makers in world health organizations and on advisory or executive boards in health ministries, regarding vaccines or in response to infectious diseases, is the "easier" course of action. As mentioned above, like lay people, experts prefer to take the easy way out rather than entering into confrontations or undermining hierarchy. Conformism, the herd mentality, and the tendency to opt for "generic" solutions, might have consequences not only for the public's trust but also for its health. Raising disputes can help to make realistic and effective decisions.

Furthermore, Sunstein argues that any decision-making process that is not accompanied by an opposing critical evaluation can lead to an extreme decision. By way of example, he cites the behavior of the U.S. Congress, stressing that the tension between the Republicans and the Democrats is necessary to avoid extreme decisions, whereas when one of the parties is weakened, the White House makes more extreme decisions.

In the realm of public health, the tendency towards universal agreement surrounding vaccines can sometimes lead to an extreme decision-making process. Examples include the aggressive marketing of the H1N1 vaccine after it was already known that the epidemic had not spread as much as expected, and administrative decisions during the Mad Cow Disease, when it was known that the British government had not regulated the meat industry properly. These are indications that falling in step with the consensus without taking other opinions into account can lead to bad decision-making.

Sunstein concludes that "organizations and nations are far more likely to prosper if they welcome dissent and promote openness. Well-functioning societies benefit from a wide range of views: their citizens do not live in gated communities or echo chambers" (2003, pp. 210–211).

### Not only exposing conflicts of interest but fighting them

It is extremely important to expose conflicts of interest but it is even more important to minimize them. Following are some ways this can be done:

1   *Extending policy makers' waiting period for applying a position in the industry* – the waiting period for policy makers before they can accept a position, receive grants or purchase stock in an industry they regulated should be extended. DeLong (2012) suggests this waiting period should be at least five years, or, ideally, ten years.

2   *Prohibition of past funding* – vaccine policy-makers, members of immunization committees and vaccine advisers should have no past funding or salaries from any vaccine companies, nor should they own stock in these companies. According to DeLong, the prohibition of past funding or salary could be phased in by setting caps on the amount a policy-maker received in the past, and lowering the caps over time, until ultimately reaching zero (DeLong, 2012).

3   *Allowing different categories of stakeholders to have a voice in decision-making regarding immunization* – in order to minimize centralization of government health authorities in immunization activities, the Israeli State Comptroller (The State Comptroller and Ombudsman of Israel, 2014) suggests allowing different categories of stakeholders, including public representatives and particularly marginalized social groups, to have a voice in decision-making, including vaccine committees. The composition of vaccine committees should include various experts, so that government health workers do not constitute a majority.

4   *Increasing transparency* – according to the Israeli State Comptroller (The State Comptroller and Ombudsman of Israel, 2014), transparency regarding the immunization policy must be increased, by providing the public full and timely information. This should include making all of the vaccine committee protocols accessible to the public.

5   *Evaluating the discussion process in the vaccine committee hearings* – To evaluate the committees' decision-making process, we must examine their protocols, discussions and documents: were all of the findings presented to them? Were dilemmas raised? Were certain subjects silenced? Who in the committee tried to promote a drug or vaccine? When? The committees must be monitored as to their decision-making processes.

6   *Conducting a study that would examine the appointment of an independent expert to coordinate the response to a threat of an outbreak* – using the case of President Obama's appointment of Ron Klain as "Ebola czar" as a study case.

7   *Communicating the vaccine committee's decisions and activities* – in order to improve the reliability of these committees.

8   *Expanding private sector involvement to include companies whose financial interests directly align with those of global health* – to ensure a balanced budgetary allocation. For example, Shah (2011) suggests that the fight against malaria should include insurance companies and tourism operators who would profit in the long run from healthier customers and less fearful tourists. Recruiting private companies like these, with health-aligned business interests, could create a wider base of private sector donors supporting the WHO, and help re-establish its authority over the global health agenda.

### Transformation of the discourse from dichotomous to complex

As mentioned, the dichotomous division made by organizations into facts versus myths, emotional versus rational, true versus false, eviscerates the purpose of scientific discourse. The organizations must transform their discourse and become self-reflective in the way they choose to present their findings to the public. The discourse with the public must take into account not only the public's concerns and fears as indicated by the risk communication research, but take another step forward and include the public in their thinking process, which will be elaborated below.

### Inclusive theoretical basis

The theoretical basis of the wisdom of crowds is that a diverse public comprised of individuals who are not experts can take certain types of decisions and make predictions just as well as experts, and in many cases even better. Tversky and Kahneman (1971) and their colleagues proved that in many cases, neither laypeople nor experts are immune to making biased, intuitive judgments. Group decision-making can happen as long as the collection of opinions comes from the biggest and most diverse group possible comprised of people with different opinions, operating in conditions of freedom of expression. Health organizations should adopt this line of thinking and pursue it in several ways: First, by creating diverse groups of experts from various disciplines with an emphasis on the communicative aspect of risk communication. Second, creating turnover between different professionals on advisory boards on epidemics and vaccines, to avoid what is known as "groupthink." Third, using the public sphere in order to apply the wisdom of crowds for assessment, planning and creativity.

### Challenges in the virtual realm

The virtual realm has created a new reality for health organizations. Social networks compose narratives that splinter and decentralize the pieces of knowledge and actually deconstruct the logocentric text of the WHO. The splintering and decentralization undermine the monolithic power field that has been held by institutions. The question is how old players will act in the new power field. As indicated, the industry tends to employ outdated commercial strategies under a new technological guise in order to promote their economic interests.

Health organizations must distinguish themselves from the industry if they want to create a real dialog with their public. They must change the methods that preserve the pattern of their scientific discourse and undergo a conceptual transformation. If they do so, they will still remain with the paradox we described in Chapter 2 of the book: engaging the public, on the one hand, and managing the information, on the other. The question is how health organizations can manage different narratives within the anarchistic tangle of the public sphere.

### Open innovation

Health is one of the top priority subjects for most digital users. Crowdsourcing (Merriam-Webster, 2015) – using social networks and digital platforms to collect information – is a well-known method. People collect information in all areas and about various issues relevant to their lifestyle. The second and more active stage of public engagement with the digital world is not only the active search of relevant information, but an attempt to receive answers to questions or problems from members of the public, not necessarily experts or doctors, and to consult not only one or two of them, but a diverse group (Zoref, 2015). Crowdsourcing can be used especially in cases where there is no simple answer, or in cases that are difficult to solve. For instance, the site www.crowdmed.com has people from all over the world trying to solve other people's complicated medical problems. The idea behind it is that in a complex world with numerous phenomena and diseases and no single doctor who can be updated about them all, this system might offer the most integrated solution. There is also a more advanced site that not only uses collective thinking to solve problems, but also offers a creative game where people seek to solve scientific problems along with experts. "Foldit" (http://fold.it/portal/) is an online puzzle video game about protein folding. The scientific game, which is constructed like a puzzle, is an attempt to crack and solve the structure of protein in order to find cures for diseases. The game has already given rise to a number of scientific breakthroughs and academic publications (Khatib et al., 2011).

The concept of "open innovation" was coined by Henry Chesbrough (2006), who described how creative ideas can be received on different subjects in order to promote products. He argues that in a complex and changing world, commercial companies cannot deal with the product on their own and must join forces, both internally within their societies, and in external partnerships with other stakeholders, "through multiple paths."

Various financial companies and intelligence communities have implemented crowdsourcing and consult a variety of experts from around the world on different issues (Global Development, 2012). In the field of health, this concept might help find solutions for complex global problems. Collaborations have been created between pharmaceutical companies, academic researchers, disease advocates and even the general public, who are drawn into the world of science through crowdsourcing (Zoref, 2015).

In an article about the concept of open innovation published in *The Guardian*, Don Joseph, chief executive of the California-based NGO BIO Ventures for Global Health, claimed that:

> The challenge is to create projects that are simple and allow a streamlined process for organizations to participate... [Open innovation partnerships could] significantly reduce trial and error, and lead neglected disease researchers to that "Eureka moment" more quickly and effectively.
> (Global Development, 2012)

If the different stakeholders join forces in the area of health, this can therefore yield the intellectual diversity and creativity that exist in the larger community. Nonetheless, the idea of crowdsourcing is still developing, and in the meantime, health organizations rely primarily on the pharmaceutical industries and on experts, and seldom consult the general public.

Health organizations can take the idea one step further, and use digital crowdsourcing to think about predicting future epidemics and addressing scientific dilemmas. The aim is to collect decentralized, varied and diverse information from all sorts of people who choose to be part of the effort, while the organization managing the epidemic crisis gathers and integrates all of the data.

A system should be designed to involve the public prior to the onset of an epidemic crisis so that it can be included in the risk communication when such a crisis does occur. The public sphere would function better as a system in times of crisis if the WHO interacts with the various publics on an ongoing basis. The culture of inclusion should be established not only during crises, but as a systemic continuum for risk communication management. Grunig and Hunt (1984), who wrote about public relations, argued that governmental organizations and authorities tend to use a one-way communication model that they have called the public information model. The aim of the communication process in this model is to inform and educate the public. Although this is an important goal, those who use it do little more than distribute information. Instead, they advocate the bidirectional symmetrical model, which, they argue, is not only the most ethical communication model, but also the most effective one (Grunig, 2001; Grunig and Huang, 2000). The aim of communication in this model is to negotiate with the public, to resolve conflicts, to better understand the audience's needs and to promote mutual understanding and respect between organizations and their publics.

Building on the observations and lessons presented above, we would like to suggest practical strategies for use particularly by local governments to stimulate engagement with the public through the social media.

## Practical Suggestions

### Goal I: Building a community presence on the social media when a crisis is imminent

Most organizations hire professionals to respond and to be present during a crisis situation. However, in order to stimulate two-way communication, there is a need to be in continual communication (not only in times of crisis) with laypeople who are active in the blogosphere and who are seen as opinion leaders – not only those who support the organizations' stance, but also those who are at odds with its policies.

The organizations should also maintain ongoing communication with experts in various fields, including not only public health experts, but also communication and sociology experts, as well as psychologists and experts in rhetoric. In addition, each country should establish continual communication with a parliament representing subgroups specific to that country. Such a parliament would promote engagement of "ordinary citizens" in discussions on policy issues in order to take into account the input of these three groups: opinion leaders, experts and citizens. Issues that do not have "scientific solutions" should be raised. As part of the parliament, a site (blog, forum) should be created to simulate two-way communication about public health concerns and possible responses. Through this "simulation forum," possible interactions between the public and government organizations can be tested with regard to various health messages and risk communicators. The messages presented to the public should be based on theoretical indexes from risk communication, including cultural sensitivity, perceptions of illness and health, questions of mistrust, rationality, dialog, inclusion, optimistic bias, uncertainty, empowerment, tailoring, and intimidation.

### Goal II: Building an automated system for identifying, monitoring and understanding social media discourse for communication in "real time"

Previous studies that used communication surveillance to analyze social media in the context of epidemic outbreaks did so from a quantitative perspective, focusing on the number of tweets and blog entries. The methodology we suggest, however, is *qualitative*, and as such, offers the possibility for a more sensitive and in-depth examination of public expression on the Internet. By identification, we do not mean identification of trends and misconceptions as health organizations usually do, but rather identification of collective memory that relates to cultural and rhetorical components.

This includes suggestions and dilemmas raised by the public, which can change even the organization's own assumptions during actual crises. The concept of crowdsourcing actually negates, as we indicated at length, the present trends of surveillance, whose purpose is to predict trends (myths, misconceptions) and debunk them. The aim is to include the public in the thinking processes and to make changes subsequent to the detection of dilemmas or ideas raised by the public.

The main questions and concerns the public raises in social media forums during pandemic outbreaks should be identified and analyzed according to the profiles of the target audiences who raise them. This stage is particularly challenging because of the segmentation of the public in a pandemic crisis. Issues that are likely to emerge include: How to account for specific language usages (for example, slang) of diverse populations? How to account for culture-specific reactions and norms of communication between members of particular groups?

In addition, an important aspect of communicating with the public during pandemic crises is the time that it takes for the media to respond to the emerging crisis. The assumption is that during health crises, the general population will turn to the media, and particularly to the Internet, to glean information (Gesser-Edelsburg, 2013). Subsequently, this stage of the project would seek to identify trends on the social media, building the groundwork for two-way communication, by enabling health organizations to respond and intervene on public media sites in real time. To facilitate this goal, the organizations should build a new and revolutionary automated system for identifying, monitoring and understanding social media trends on the social networks during crises. In addition, local organizations should establish an automatic risk communication system based on preliminary risk communication simulations with representatives of different groups within the public.

### Goal III: Emergency knowledge management system

Based on the analysis of social media trends, social media communication content analysis and sentiment analysis, a primary goal of health organizations should be to create an emergency knowledge management system that brings together the input of public discourse in social media with the action/response of emergency agencies, in order to create effective interaction between them. Disaster response requires coordinated central responses and actions in real time. Crisis management software can be used to organize the information into functional areas, an important task as information arrives piecemeal from different sources. Instead of a traditional collaborative system based on face-to-face meetings of representatives of various agencies, information should be gathered and centralized in one system. This is an ongoing process that takes into account the different events routinely occurring. The aim is to create a technological system that considers and is informed by input from the public and government agencies in order to build a unified knowledge base to coordinate, adjust, improve and document the interaction between all sides, ensuring ever-growing efficacy.

In the digital age, organizations can deconstruct what Foucault called the field of knowledge/power by using the different narratives of diverse publics to create a more balanced democratic system that also has creative flexibility. For that to happen, the establishment must change its mode of thinking in its scientific discourse, while at the same time building digital and communication systems that use crowdsourcing to solve scientific problems, and involving and including the public in the discourse in the public sphere. These steps can contribute to a different risk management approach for epidemic crises, bringing organizations closer to their metaphorical potential of embracing the public sphere.

## References

Baron, R. S., and Kerr, N. L. (2003). *Group Process, Group Decision, Group Action* (2nd Edition). Buckingham: Open University Press.

Chesbrough, H. W. (2006). *Open Business Models: How to Thrive in the New Innovation Landscape.* Boston: Harvard Business School Press.

DeLong, G. (2012). Conflicts of interest in vaccine safety research. *Accountability in Research*, 19(2), 65–88.

ECDC. (2012). *Communication on Immunisation – Building Trust.* Stockholm: European Centre for Disease Prevention and Control.

Foucault, M. (1981). The order of things: An archaeology of the human sciences. In R. J. C. Young (Ed.), *Untying the Text: A Post-structuralist Reader* (pp. 48–78). London: Routledge and Kegan Paul.

Gesser-Edelsburg, A. (2013). Strategies for communicating with the public effectively using websites and social media during emergencies and disease outbreaks. In M. S. Green and E. Mordini (Eds.), *Internet-Based Intelligence for Public Health Emergencies and Disease Outbreak: Technical, Medical and Regulatory Issues* (pp. 73–83). Amsterdam: IOS Press BV.

Global Development. (2012). Crowdsourcing reveals life-saving potential in global health research. *The Guardian.* August 15. Available at: www.theguardian.com/global-development/2012/aug/15/crowdsourcing-global-health-research

Grunig, J. E. (2001). Two-way symmetrical public relations: Past, present, and future. In R. L. Heath and G. M. Vasques (Eds.), *Handbook of Public Relations* (pp. 11–30). Newbury Park, CA: Sage.

Grunig, J. E., and Huang, Y. H. (2000). From organizational effectiveness to relationship indicators: Antecedents of relationships, public relations strategies, and relationship outcomes. In J. A. Ledingham and S. D. Bruning (Eds.), *Public Relations as Relationship Management: A Relational Approach to the Study and Practice of Public Relations* (pp. 23–54). Mahwah, NJ: Lawrence Erlbaum Associates.

Grunig, J. E., and Hunt, T. (1984). *Managing Public Relations* New York: Holt, Rinehart and Winston.

Jehn, K. A. (1995). A multimethod examination of the benefits and detriments of intragroup conflict. *Administrative Science Quarterly*, 40(2), 256–282.

Jehn, K. A., Northcraft, G. B., and Neale, M. A. (1999). Why differences make a difference: A field study of diversity, conflict and performance in workgroups. *Administrative Science Quarterly*, 44(4), 741–763.

Khatib, F., DiMaio, F., Cooper, S., *et al.* (2011). Crystal structure of a monomeric retroviral protease solved by protein folding game players. *Nature Structural and Molecular Biology*, 18(10), 1175–1177.

Loury, G. C. (1994). Self-censorship in public discourse: A theory of "political correctness" and related phenomena. *Rationality and Society*, 6(4), 428–461.

Lyon, T. P., and Maxwell, J. W. (2004). Astroturf: Interest group lobbying and corporate strategy. *Journal of Economics and Management Strategy*, 13(4), 561–597.

Merriam-Webster. (2015). Definition of crowdsourcing. Available at: www.merriam -webster.com/dictionary/crowdsourcing (accessed May 20, 2016).

Mills, S. (2003). *Michel Foucault*. London: Routledge.

Oreskes, N., and Conway, E. M. (2011). *Merchants of Doubt: How a Handful of Scientists Obscured the Truth on Issues from Tobacco Smoke to Global Warming*. New York: Bloomsbury Press.

Shah, S. (2011). How private companies are transforming the global public health agenda: A new era for the World Health Organization. *Foreign Affairs*, November 9.

Sunstein, C. R. (2003). *Why Societies Need Dissent*. Cambridge, MA: Harvard University Press.

Surowiecki, J. (2005). *The Wisdom of Crowds: Why the Many Are Smarter Than the Few*. New York: Anchor Books.

The State Comptroller and Ombudsman of Israel. (2014). *The Immunization Set for Children, Adults and Medical Staff. Annual Report 64c*. Available at: www.mevaker. gov.il/he/Reports/Report_248/c51ffb79-e3a9-49b3-9654-8054462506ba/214-ver-4.pdf (In Hebrew) (accessed April 26, 2016).

The White House. (2009). Remarks by the President at the National Academy of Sciences annual meeting. April 27. Retrieved from https://www.whitehouse.gov/the-press-office/ remarks-president-national-academy-sciences-annual-meeting.

Tversky, A., and Kahneman, D. (1971). Belief in the law of small numbers. *Psychological Bulletin*, 76(2), 105–110.

Zoref, L. (2015). *Mindsharing: The Art of Crowdsourcing Everything*. New York: Penguin Publishing Group.

# Index